DEVELOPMENTS IN DRUGS USED IN ANAESTHESIA

BOERHAAVE SERIES
FOR POSTGRADUATE
MEDICAL EDUCATION
Vol. 23

PROCEEDINGS OF BOERHAAVE COURSES
ORGANIZED BY
THE FACULTY OF MEDICINE, UNIVERSITY OF LEIDEN
THE NETHERLANDS

For complete series listing please refer to the last page in this book

DEVELOPMENTS IN DRUGS USED IN ANAESTHESIA

edited by

J. SPIERDIJK M.D.
Department of Anaesthesiology, Leiden University Hospital,
Leiden

S.A. FELDMAN M.D.
Department of Anaesthetics, Westminster Hospital,
London

H. MATTIE M.D.
Department of Clinical Pharmacology, Leiden University Hospital,
Leiden

T.H. STANLEY M.D.
Department of Anaesthesiology, College of Medicine,
Salt Lake City

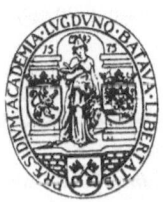

1981
SPRINGER-SCIENCE+BUSINESS MEDIA, B.V.

ISBN 978-94-009-7974-1   ISBN 978-94-009-7972-7 (eBook)
DOI 10.1007/978-94-009-7972-7

CONTENTS

CONTRIBUTORS

S. Agoston, Department of Anaesthesiology, University Hospital, Groningen, The Netherlands.

A. Atinault, Department of Physiology, Research Institute for Electrical Anaesthesia Faculty of Dental Surgery, Montrouge, France.

L. Barritault, Department of Physiology, Research Institute for Electrical Anaesthesia, Faculty of Dental Surgery, Montrouge, France.

J.G. Bovill, Department of Anaesthesiology, University Hospital, Amsterdam,The Netherlands.

D.D. Breimer, Department of Pharmacology, Subfaculty of Pharmacy, Leyden University, Sylvius Laboratory, Leyden, The Netherlands.

J.B. Cazalaa, Department of Physiology, Research Institute for Electrical Anaesthesia, Faculty of Dental Surgery, Montrouge, France.

B.F. Cohn, Department of Anaesthesiology, University Hospital, Leyden, The Netherlands.

C.M. Conway, Magill Department of Anaesthesiology, Westminster Hospital, London U.K.

J.T. Davidson, Department of Anaesthesia, Hadassah University Hospital, Jerusalem, Israel.

A. Doenicke, Department of Anaesthesia, University Hospital,Munchen, Germany.

Th. Duka, Department of Anaesthesia, University Hospital,Munchen, Germany.

E.I. Eger, Department of Anaesthesiology, University of California, San Francisco, California, U.S.A.

S.A. Feldman, President of the International College of Anaesthetists, Department of Anaesthesiology, Westminster Hospital, London U.K.

W. Flameng, Department of Cardiovascular Surgery, University Hospital, Leuven, Belgium.

P. Janssen, Janssen Pharmaceutica, Beerse, Belgium.

J.W. van Kleef, Department of Anaesthesiology, University Hospital, Leyden, The Netherlands.

D.W. Koopman, Department of Anaesthesiology, University Hospital, Leyden The Netherlands.

S. de Lange, Department of Anaesthesiology, University Hospital, Leyden, The Netherlands.

A. Limoge, Department of Physiology, Research Institute for Electrical Anaesthesia, Faculty of Dental Surgery, Montrouge, France.

Y. Louville, Department of Physiology, Research Institute for Electrical Anaesthesia, Faculty of Dental Surgery, Montrouge, France.

H. Mattie, Department of Clinical Pharmacology, University Hospital Leyden, The Netherlands.

D.C. Moore, Department of Anaesthesiology, The Mason Clinic, Seattle, Washington, U.S.A.

J.H. Nauta, Department of Anaesthesiology, University Hospital, Leyden, The Netherlands.

P. Rog, Department of Anaesthesiology, University Hospital, Amsterdam, The Netherlands.

G. Rolly, Department of Anaesthesiology, University Hospital, Gent, Belgium.

P.S. Sebel, Department of Anaesthesiology, University Hospital,
Amsterdam, The Netherlands.

W. Soudijn, Department of Pharmaceutical Chemistry, University of Amsterdam, Amsterdam, The Netherlands.

Joh. Spierdijk, Department of Anaesthesiology, University Hospital, Leyden,
The Netherlands.

Th.H. Stanley, Department of Anaesthesiology, College of Medicine, Salt
Lake City, Utah, U.S.A.

N. Ty Smith, Department of Anaesthesiology, University of California,
San Diego, Veterans Administration Hospital, San Diego, California,U.S.A.

L. Versichelen, Department of Anaesthesiology, University Hospital, Gent,
Belgium.

A. Wauquier, Department of Pharmacology, Janssen Pharmaceutica,
Beerse, Belgium.

A. Witter, Rudolf Magnus Instituut, University of Utrecht, Utrecht,
The Netherlands.

N.A. Zubair, Department of Anaesthesiology, University Hospital, Gent,
Belgium.

PREFACE

This book reflects the proceedings of the Boerhaave Course,
"Developments in drugs used in Anaesthesia", held on May 7th and 8th
1981 at Leiden University.

The goal of the organizers of the course was to obtain a better understanding of the pharmacological and clinical applications of the drugs
used in the field of Anaesthesiology. In my opinion, there is a constant
need for post-graduate teaching not only on a clinical basis, but also
in the so-called "basic sciences". This especially applies to
anaesthetists.

I would like to express my thanks to the speakers, who were all so
kind as to send their manuscripts in time for publishing, and to thank
the co-editors of this book, as well as Mr. B.F. Commandeur, from Mar-
tinus Nijhoff Publishers for their fruitful co-operation. Last but not
least, I would like to thank the secretarial staff of my department
for all the work they did arranging for manuscripts to be in the right
places at the right times.

Joh. Spierdijk

THE USE OF H$_2$ BLOCKERS

T.H. STANLEY

In the last decade a new important histamine receptor, H$_2$ receptor, has been discovered which has major importance in gastric acid production. In addition, a new drug Cimetidine (Tagamet) which blocks the H$_2$ receptor has been synthesized. The object of this presentation will be to discuss the possible role of this interesting drug (Cimetidine) before and during operation and possible postoperatively as well.

There is, as many of you know, a disease entity called Mendelson's syndrome which does not occur frequently but when it does can produce severe pulmonary embarrassment and death in anesthetized patients.[1-7] Mendelson's syndrome or pulmonary acid aspiration, as it is more commonly called occurs when gastric contents with a pH of less than 2.5 is aspirated into the lungs. It appears that gastric juice with a pH >2.5 does not produce changes in the lung (which, incidentally, include hemorrhage, edema, and cellular and structural damage and result in hypoxia). It also appears that a critical volume of gastric juice (0.4 ml/kg or< 25 ml) as well as a pH of<2.5 is necessary for the production of this syndrome.

The actual incidence of pulmonary acid aspiration in the surgical patient is unknown as it may occur as a subclinical problem manifesting itself as postoperative pneumonia, atelectasis or intraoperative or postoperative pulmonary dysfunction of unknown etiology. It is known, however, that certain anesthetics may increase the risk of this problem by increasing gastric acid production while others decrease this risk by doing the opposite. There is also evidence that premedication, especially heavy premedication, may reduce the risk of acid aspiration by decreasing acid production.

Other factors that increase the risk of pulmonary acid inspiration include patients who for whatever reason have a large volume of gastric fluid, patients with hiatus hernia with reflux, the presence of passive regurgitation, patient positions that promote reflux or regurgitation, and failure to fast preoperatively.

In recent years attempts have been made, especially in the pregnant patient about to undergo anesthesia (a patient population most especially at risk of sustaining acid pulmonary aspiration because of delayed gastric emptying) to reduce both gastric volume and pH. The first drug group studied were the anticholinergic drugs (atropine, scopolamine). While these drugs can reduce gastric juice volume, their effects are quite variable. In addition, they have little influence on gastric pH and decrease gastric emptying and esophageal tone, both of which increase the risk of gastric reflux. Another undesirable effect of the anticholinergics is that heart rate is increased.

A second drug studied recently is glycopyrrolate. This compound reduces gastric volume and increases pH but it, like the anticholinergics, is not fool-proof. A recent study comparing glycopyrrolate, atropine, and patients receiving no drug (control) demonstrated that neither drug significantly altered the mean pH or volume of gastric juice in preoperative patients nor reduced the incidence of patients with gastric juice pH below 2.5.

Antacids have also been used to neutralize acid gastric juice contents in patients about to undergo operation but while they do increase pH they also increase gastric volume and thus increase the risk of reflux. Antacids possess the additional disadvantages of causing pulmonary damage themselves (when aspirated) and requiring administration at least 30 minutes before induction of anesthesia for effectiveness.

A couple of recently performed studies have indicated that while acid injection into the lung produces dramatic increases in pulmonary hemorrhage, exudates and edema and alkaline solutions produce no histologic changes (although they do increase pulmonary shunting) antacids produce bronchopneumonia. Thus, seemingly innocuous drugs may not be innocuous at all when aspirated into the lungs.

For many years you have heard how gastric acid is increased with histamine, gastric acid and acetylcholine. You've also heard about H_2 receptors and how histamine stimulates these receptors and Cimetidine blocks them. This all suggests that Cimetidine may be effective in acid pulmonary aspiration by decreasing acid production and gastric volume and thus decreasing the incidence and magnitude of pulmonary damage, should aspiration occur.

Initial studies done with oral Cimetidine (400 mg) administered with preoperative premedicants indicated that the percent of patients with gastric pH above 2.5 was markedly increased over controls for up to 6-8 hours. Unfortunately, gastric volume was not significantly altered with this therapy. Another study demonstrated that oral Cimetidine only given immediately before operation is ineffective in increasing pH and reducing gastric volume. However, oral Cimetidine given the night before and immediately before operation does increase gastric pH. In the latter study the best regimen was either intramuscular or intravenous Cimetidine which both reduced gastric volume as well as increased gastric pH. Of the latter, IV therapy was best as it acted sooner and produced the most dramatic results. However, giving IV Cimetidine as routine preoperative medication is cumbersome in most hopsitals and as a result therapy employing Cimetidine orally at the hour of sleep the night before operation and IM just before operation seems equally effective. One study has demonstrated that this therapy is better than no Cimetidine, oral Cimetidine the morning of surgery or oral Cimetidine the night before and morning of operation.

Intravenous Cimetidine is gaining popularity in open heart surgery and in intensive care units to reduce G.I. bleeding secondary to gastric acid production. Preliminary findings (de Lange,3.,unpublished data) indicate the compound has little effect on cardiovascular dynamics when given intravenously either before or during operation.

The infrequently occurring adverse effects of Cimetidine which have only been reported in a few patients receiving chronic, higher dose Cimetidine have not been found when the drug is given either before or during anesthesia (Stanley TH, unpublished data).

Thus, Cimetidine is a good compound to use in the pre or intraoperative period to reduce gastric volume and increase pH and should reduce the incidence and magnitude of acid pulmonary aspiration. It appears that IV is better than IM usage but that a combination of oral Cimetidine at the hour of sleep and IM preoperatively about one hour before operation will work fine in almost everyone.

REFERENCES

1. Husemeyer RP, Davenport HT, Rajasekaran T: Cimetidine as a single oral dose for prophylaxis against Mendelson's syndrome. Anaesthesia 33:775-778, 1978.
2. Keating PJ, Black JF, Watson DW: Effects of glycopyrolate and Cimetidine on gastric volume and acidity in patients awaiting surgery. Br J Anaesth 50:1247-1249, 1978.
3. Weber LA, Kirschman CA: Cimetidine for prophylaxis of aspiration pneumonitis: Comparison of intramuscular and oral dosage schedules. Anesthesiology 51: S180, 1979.
4. Coombs DW, Hooper D, Cotton T: Acid-aspiration prophylaxis by use of preoperative oral administration of cimetidine. Anesthesiology 51: 352-355, 1979.
5. Stoelting RK: Gastric fluid pH in patients receiving cimetidine. Anesth Analg 57:675-677, 1978.
6. Coombs DW, Hooper D, Cotton T: Pre-anesthetic cimetine for alteration of gastric fluid volume and pH. Anesth Analg 58:183-188, 1979.
7. Teabeaut JR: Aspiration of gastric contents: An experimental study. Am J Pathol 28:51-67, 1975.

GENERAL PHARMACOKINETIC PRINCIPLES OF INDUCTION AGENTS

D.D. BREIMER

Department of Pharmacology, Subfaculty of Pharmacy, University of Leiden.

INTRODUCTION

Drugs produce their pharmacological effect in biological systems by reacting with receptor sites, which are located in the target tissues. The intensity of effect of reversibly acting drugs depends on the degree of receptor occupation, which, in turn, is determined by the concentration of the drug in the direct environment of the receptors (biophase) and the affinity of the drug for the receptors. Usually, it is not possible to determine drug concentrations at the receptor sites in man, since these are not accessible for sampling. However, all tissues are supplied with plasma and it is obvious that a certain relationship must exist between drug concentration in plasma and the concentration in the biophase, although such a relationship may be complex. The plasma is easily accessible for sampling. Following the administration of a drug to man or animal, several processes take place: 1. absorption from the site of application to the plasma; 2. distribution from the plasma into organs and tissues, and 3. elimination by biotransformation (e.g. in the liver) or by excretion (e.g. through the kidney). As a consequence of these events, which partly occur simultaneously, the drug concentration in plasma changes with time. Likewise, the concentration in the biophase also changes and so does the pharmacological effect. In other words, changes in the time course of drug concentrations in plasma will affect the time course of drug action. It is for this reason that information on the kinetics of a drug in the body is of great interest for clinical practice in general and for anaesthesiology in particular. In anaesthesiology many drugs are being applied and their onset and duration of

action is one of the key features during operation. Pharmacokinetic data
will help to optimize drug application, with respect to the choice of
the appropriate drug and drug preparation, as well as with respect to a
proper dosage regimen.

PHARMACOKINETICS AND PHARMACOKINETIC MODELS

Pharmacokinetics deals with the kinetics of absorption, distribution,
metabolism and excretion of drugs and other substances in man or animals.
Its purpose is to study the time course of drug concentrations in plasma
and other fluids, tissues and excreta and to construct models suitable
to interpret such data. The relationship between pharmacological response
and concentrations of drugs or their metabolites in body fluids is also
pertinent to pharmacokinetics. Several textbooks and reviews have
recently been published in the area of pharmacokinetics and clinical
pharmacokinetics (1 - 4).

One of the basic tools of science is the use of models to simulate
and simplify real systems. In physiology and pharmacokinetics compartment
models are often used to describe the behaviour of endogenous substances
or exogenous substances, including drugs, although recently also more
physiological models are being applied (1). Compartmental models assume
that the biological system can be described as one or more connected
pools, in which an amount of drug may be homogeneously distributed
throughout an apparent volume of distribution. The transfer of drug
between compartments is usually assumed to proceed by an apparent first-
order process. In Fig. 1 a representation is given of the processes
taking place after administration of a drug to the body. These involve
consecutive and simultaneous competing rate processes or clearance
processes, where clearance may be thought of as that volume of the
total volume of a certain compartment which is totally cleared of drug
per unit of time. Compartment O may for instance, represent the g.i.
tract after oral administration of a drug and to the central compartment
belong the plasma, blood cells, and the well-perfused organs and tissues.
Additionally it may be distinguished between a peripheral compartment
and a brain compartment which, for i.v. induction agents, includes the

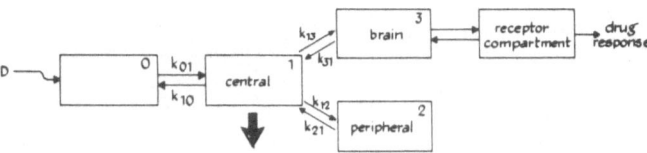

FIGURE 1. In this theoretical schema a representation is given of the various rate processes taking place in the body after administration of a drug. The k-symbols represent the rate or clearance constants to and from the various compartments. The heavy arrow from the central compartment indicates the elimination process of the drug from the body, either by excretion or by biotransformation or by a combination of both.

the receptors. The heavy arrow from the central compartment represents the elimination process of the drug from the body via the kidney (water soluble or hydrophilic compounds like induction agents) or via the lungs (volatile agents like many general anaesthetic drugs). This model on paper looks rather complex and although it may even be realistic, it should be realized that in practice the possibility of determining drug concentrations will generally be limited to the central or plasma compartment. In other words we generally are only able, at least in humans, to measure plasma concentrations and from these it is often rather difficult or impossible to extrapolate to the absolute concentration in certain discrete areas of the body. With regard to the concentration time-course in the various parts of the body it may, however, be somewhat simpler, if one assumes that after a certain time a distribution equilibrium is established between the various compartments, so that the concentration decay in every compartment ultimately parallels the

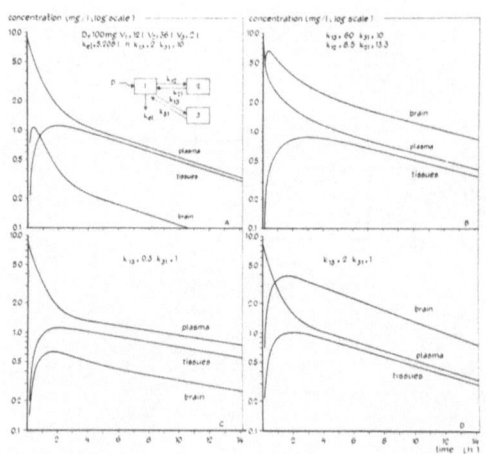

FIGURE 2.   *Theoretical curves representing drug concentration in plasma and tissues rapidly equilibrating with plasma (compartment 1), the other tissues of the body (compartment 2) and the brain (compartment 3). The pharmacokinetic parameters underlying these curves are given in A. and B. The clearance constants governing drug entry into the brain (k_{13}) and from the brain (k_{31}) are varied and the influence on the brain concentration and on the concentrations in the other two compartments is shown. The brain concentration may vary considerably despite comparable plasma concentrations.*

the decay in plasma. Examples of such situations are given in Fig. 2, following rapid i.v. administration of drugs (directly into compartment 1) with different distribution characteristics. Compartment 2 represents a peripheral one and compartment 3 the brain. The values for the rate of brain penetration have been varied and it can be seen that only if brain penetration is rapid, immediately after drug administration high brain concentrations are achieved, which further closely follow the concentration in plasma. Such a situation is likely to be representative for thiopental and other induction agents following i.v. injection. This will be discussed in more detail later. If brain penetration is slower, then lower brain concentrations are reached which makes a rapid onset of CNS action less likely to occur.

The other important feature that can be deduced from Fig. 2 is that the plasma concentration time course following i.v. injection of a drug very often shows two distinct phases: an initial rapid decay (distribution phase), during which predominantly distribution takes place into the other compartments and a second slower decay, which represents the elimination phase. From such curves parameters like distribution and elimination half-lives can be deduced, as well as total body clearance. Furthermore the volumes of distribution can be calculated.

PHARMACOKINETICS OF INDUCTION AGENTS

General requirements

Drugs used to induce anaesthesia are required to have a rapid onset of action following i.v. administration and preferably also a short and predictable duration of action. Such properties are the result of certain rather specific pharmacological, physico-chemical and pharmacokinetic characteristics of an i.v. anaesthetic.

The onset of drug action is dependent on the rate of drug administration and the rate of brain penetration; only highly lipophilic compounds will distribute into and throughout the brain very rapidly. The duration of anaesthetic action of most induction agents is primarily dependent on the dose administered and the rate of redistribution of the drug from well perfused tissues (brain) to less well perfused tissues; the duration of residual effects are often determined by the rate of elimination (biotransformation) of the compound from the body. These aspects will further be discussed and illustrated in the following section. The kinetic processes of drug distribution and drug elimination are generally studied on the basis of plasma concentration time curves, from which a number of important pharmacokinetic parameters can be deduced (e.g. elimination half-life, volume of distribution, total body clearance). For most induction agents used in clinical practice the average values of these parameters are known and some examples are given in Table I. The pharmacokinetics of some these

TABLE I. Average values of elimination half-lives ($t_{\frac{1}{2}}$) apparent volumes of distribution (V_d) and clearance of some induction agents following i.v. administration

Compound	$t_{\frac{1}{2}}$ (h)	V_d (1/kg)	Clearance (ml/min)	Reference
Thiopental	6.2	1.6	144	24
Methohexital	1.6	1.1	825	8
Ketamine	3.4	3.3	1296	25
Etomidate	3.5	3.7	879	26
Flunitrazepam	22	4.1	130	27
Midazolam	2.1	1.1	462	28

drugs have recently extensively been reviewed (5, 6).

Drug distribution and duration of anaesthetic action

The pharmacokinetics of an induction agent in relation to its onset and duration of anaesthetic effect will be discussed briefly, by taking the widely studied compound thiopental as an example. A single i.v. injection of thiopental (about 3-4 mg/kg) produces loss of consciousness within 10 sec and a state of anaesthesia that lasts for about 3 to 5 min. The drug is very lipid soluble and penetrates through the blood brain barrier very rapidly. Since the brain receives a relatively large proportion of cardiac output, also a large proportion of the drug will get into the brain quickly. However, the concentration of thiopental in the blood rapidly decreases as a result of distribution of the drug into other well-perfused tissues. Consequently also brain concentration decreases rapidly again, because the high lipid solubility of the compound also means rapid rate of exit from the brain. Redistribution to muscle tissue is most probably the major reason for the ultrashort action of thiopental following single i.v. injection. In hypovolaemia the blood flow to muscle is reduced and blood supply to brain and heart is maintained. This will result in higher and longer lastingly high concentrations in brain and heart, which causes marked cerebral and cardiac depression of longer duration than under normal conditions (5).

It is important to realize that the rate of redistribution of thiopental, and most probably of other induction agents as well, is responsible for the desired short duration of anaesthetic action. Drug elimination plays only a minor role during this period, in particular if total body clearance is low (Table I). However, on repeated administration of for instance thiopental, at relatively short intervals, the rate of drug elimination may become a decisive factor in the duration of anaesthetic action. Drug accumulation occurs and after some time a situation is reached in which drug concentration remains above the threshold for anaesthetic response, not only during the rapidly declining distribution phase, but also partially during the elimination phase. Hence a disproportionate increase in duration of anaesthetic action will occur. Such a situation is less likely to happen with rapidly eliminated induction agents (those with a high clearance, Table I).

Drug elimination and duration of residual effects

It is desirable that induction agents not only exhibit a short duration of anaesthetic effect, but also a short duration of post-anaesthetic CNS depressant or residual effects. The latter is predominantly determined by the rate of elimination of drug from the body, which for induction agents occurs by biotransformation in the liver. Following thiopental administration residual effects occur for a relatively long time, which is most probably due to its relative slow rate of metabolism, although also ultimate redistribution from adipose tissue may become a rate-determining step for its elimination. In any case the disappearance rate from plasma is a decisive factor in the duration of effect for thiopental, as was illustrated in a comparitive investigation in large domestic animals (7). In cattle, sheep, goats and swine thiopental caused anaesthesia of short duration. However, after regaining consciousness residual CNS depressant effects lasted very long in cattle, whereas this was far shorter in the other animal species (Table II). It appeared that in all species the initial distribution phase in the plasma concentration time curve was rapid, but the elimination phase was by far the slowest in cattle. This situation is compared for cattle and sheep   in Fig. 3.

TABLE II. *Response of animals to thiopental after a single i.v.*
injection of the drug (7).

Species	Dose (mg/kg)	Duration of anaesthesia (min)	Duration of residual CNS depression (hr)
Cattle	20	32.25 + 14.36	19.25 + 2.63
Sheep	20	18.30 + 5.10	0.8 + 0.3
Goats	12.7 - 13.9	12.00 + 5.20	0.6 + 0.1

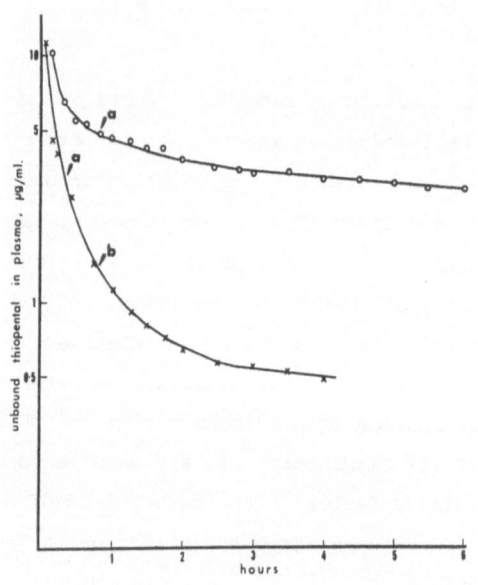

FIGURE 3. *Plasma disappearance of thiopental in cattle (o) and sheep*
(x) after an identical dose (20 mg/kg). Each value represents an average
of four animals. The pointers indicate regain of consciousness (a) and
disappearance of residual CNS depressant effects (b) respectively. In
cattle, the latter phase lasted for more than 19 hr (7).

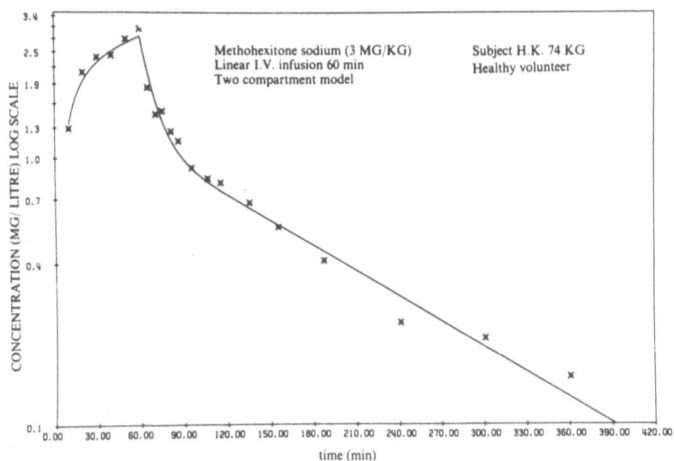

FIGURE 4. Plasma concentration curve of methohexital during and after a 60-min zero-order i.v. infusion (3 mg/kg) into a healthy volunteer. The elimination half-life of methohexital in this subject was 95 min as deduced from the terminal linear part of the curve (8).

In contrast to thiopental, the other commonly used barbiturate for i.v. anaesthesia, methohexital, is very rapidly metabolized in humans (half-life of elimination between 1 and 2 h) (8). Complete recovery with absence of residual effects seems to occur significantly more rapid following methohexital than following thiopental administration (9), which is in agreement with its rapid rate of bioinactivation. In Fig. 4 the plasma concentration time curve of methohexital is shown, during and following slow i.v. infusion of the drug to a healthy volunteer. After infusion the characteristic distribution phase (rapid decay) and elimination phase (slower decay) can be distinguished.

In general a rapid rate of elimination of an induction agent is of advantage in clinical practice and pharmacokinetic parameters like elimination half-life and total clearance (Table I) are to be regarded as important - but not the only - criteria for making a proper choice. Similar considerations apply in the case of hypnotic drugs, of which it is desirable that the duration of action is restricted to the night. The next morning hangover effects and residual impairment of performance should be absent and therefore relatively short-acting hypnotics are to be preferred. However, only few barbiturates or benzodiazepines have short elimination half-lives and the ones most commonly applied are relatively long-acting which is in agreement with their slow elimination rate (10, 11).

Drug infusion and continuous effect

During some operations anaesthesia is to be maintained with an i.v. induction agent, which means that the drug has to be administered by i.v. infusion. Of course, first a rapid i.v. injection has to be given in order to produce anaesthesia and subsequently relatively high plasma concentrations are maintained by continuing drug administration with zero-order infusion. It is important to realize that real constant plasma concentrations are only reached after about 4 times the elimination half-life of the drug and that the height of this constant concentration (steady-state) is determined by total clearance only (1 - 5). This implies that this is in fact only feasible in anaesthesia with drugs that have short elimination half-lives and are rapidly cleared. Duration of anaesthesia is now in fact determined by the equilibrium between rate of infusion and the rate of drug elimination and not by drug distribution as is the case following single dose injection. After stopping infusion recovery will be rapid if indeed the drug is rapidly inactivated. Experiments with etomidate have shown that it is possible to maintain anaesthesia by infusing this drug and still regain consciousness relatively rapidly after operation (12, 13).

INTERINDIVIDUAL VARIABILITY IN PHARMACOKINETICS

There is wide variability among patients in their response to the same dose of a drug. Much of this interindividual variability can be explained by pharmacokinetic factors: absorption, distribution, biotransformation or metabolism and excretion. The rate of these processes for a given drug is influenced by many factors pertaining to pathophysiological circumstances, to genetic variables (in particular those determing drug metabolism), to the age and diet of the patient, to effects caused by other drugs taken concurrently, etc. In many instances, and in particular with drugs having a small therapeutic ratio, drug dosage must be individualized if the desired response with minimal side effects is to be obtained. Since the effect of drugs is often better correlated with plasma concentrations than with the given dose, the measurement of drug plasma concentrations can be very helpful in the management of individual drug therapy. This is often done for drugs which are given chronically and for which the therapeutic concentration range has been established (anti-epileptic drugs, anti-arrhytmic drugs and others) (14). In anaesthetic practice it is not very feasible to monitor drug concentrations during operation, but it is important to consider and take into account the various factors which cause that one patient differs widely from the other in response to an induction agent. Of course also differences in receptor sensitivity will play a role in this respect, but only pharmacokinetic factors will be briefly reviewed here. For a more extensive review the reader is referred to other literature sources (15, 16).

Drug absorption

In anaesthesia most drugs are given by injection, so that absorption of drugs from the gastrointestinal tract is beyond the scope of this chapter. Sometimes absorption from the site of intramuscular injection to the blood may be relatively slow, which causes delayed onset of drug action. Such slow absorption is probably associated with a super-ficial injection technique and/or decreased tissue perfusion. In this regard the results of an interesting investigation are shown in Fig. 5; diazepam was given i.m. by doctors and nurses and the plasma concen-trations at 90 min following injection were compared. There is wide variability and generally doctors seem to inject more efficiently than nurses.

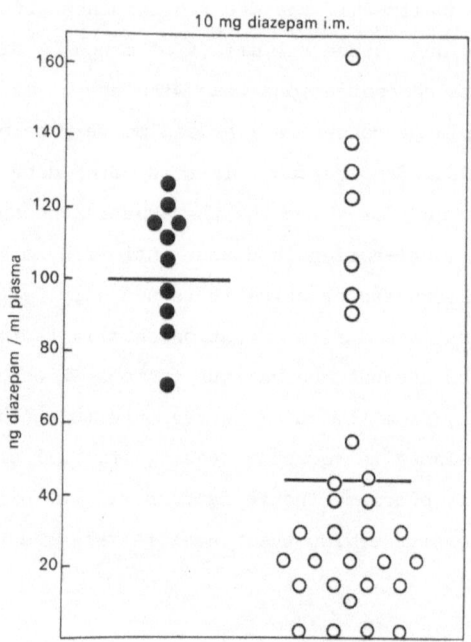

FIGURE 5. Diazepam concentrations in plasma at 90 min following intra-muscular injection of 10 mg diazepam to hospitalized patients: left, injection given by doctors; right, injection given by nurses (23).

Drug distribution

Once the drug is in the blood stream it will further quickly distribute over the various organs and tissues. The extent and rate at which this occurs is dependent on the following factors, which may vary considerably from one individual to the other:

- body weight;
- body composition (e.g. adipose versus muscle tissues);
- cardiac output and blood flow to the various organs and tissues;
- binding to plasma proteins (albumin concentrations, interactions);
- tissue binding.

First of all body weight is mentioned, since it seems obvious that in a patient with a relatively low body weight, higher concentrations are to be expected in plasma and tissues than in a patient with a relatively high body weight when the same dose of a drug is given to both patients. This factor is often not taken into account in drug therapy, partially because of the many practical difficulties involved to do otherwise. However, in anaesthesia and also in pediatrics drug dosage is often adjusted to body weight or body surface.

Body composition may vary considerably; for instance with increasing age adipose tissue tends to increase at the expense of functional tissue like muscles. Also in the elderly body-water and albumin concentration are decreased, as well as cardiac output, splanchnic blood flow and renal blood flow (17). These events may influence the onset and duration of induction agents considerably, because - as was outlined previously - drug distribution and redistribution are decisive factors in this respect. They at least partially explain the higher sensitivity of agents like thiopental in the elderly.

An important factor in drug distribution is the binding to plasma proteins, in particular albumin. Only the unbound fraction is freely available for distribution into tissues and thereby available to receptor sites, but also to elimination sites. Protein binding varies between patients and is particularly sensitive to certain diseases which are associated with decreased albumin (e.g. liver cirrhosis) or an increase of bound endogenous substances like bilirubin (e.g. hepatitis).

Disease states which do not primarily affect protein binding may be important with respect to drug distribution. For instance in myocardial infarction, complicated by shock, or in heart failure, the apparent volumes of distribution of lidocaine and procainamide were found to be reduced, probably owing to the reduced blood supply to peripheral tissues. This results in higher plasma concentrations and unexpected toxicity. A similar finding was noted in patients with acute viral hepatitis, who showed increased drug sensitivity to hexobarbital during i.v. infusion. In these patients the concentration during infusion rose more rapidly than in healthy controls, which could not be explained by the reduced rate of metabolism during this short period of time. The initial distribution volume was found to be significantly reduced in these patients (18).

Renal excretion

Hydrophilic drugs or metabolites are eliminated from the body by renal excretion, which is dependent upon the net consequence of glomerular filtration, tubular secretion and tubular reabsorption. Patients with renal insufficiency exhibit a decreased urinary excretion rate of renally cleared compounds and these will show a prolonged elimination half-life. If dosage is not adjusted accumulation into the toxic concentration range will become manifest during chronic drug therapy, as is the case for digoxin, aminoglycoside antibiotics and others. For some of these clin- ically very important drugs it has been shown that a linear relationship exists between creatinine clearance and the elimination rate constant of the drug. Based upon this relationship the dosage of drugs can be adjusted in renal insufficiency and also in the elderly with reduced renal capacity.

Drug metabolism

Lipophilic drugs (e.g. i.v. induction agents) are metabolized by drug metabolizing enzymes in the liver, which generally renders them more hydrophilic and hence they can be excreted as metabolites in urine. Interindividual differences in the rate of drug metabolism represents the major cause of interindividual variability in pharmacokinetics. For example the elimination half-life of diazepam among healthy adults varies from 9 to 53 h. It should be realized that the elimination half-life of a drug is also influenced by the volume of distribution, but it is in particular the rate of metabolism (metabolic clearance) that is responsible for such manifold variation. This is due to the fact that drug metabolizing enzyme activity is influenced by many factors:

- genetic factors;
- age and sex;
- environmental factors(exposure to chemicals, smoking);
- diet;
- disease (liver disease, thyroid disease);
- interactions with other drugs (inhibition, induction).

Genetic factors play a very important role in drug metabolism and clear polymorphism has been shown to exist for instance for N-acetylation

of isoniazid, hydralazine, procainamide. A similar phenomenon is encountered in the hydrolysis of suxamethonium and in the oxidation of the anti-
hypertensive agent debrisoquine.

With increasing age there is a tendency that drug metabolizing activity
decreases, although this is surely not true for every drug (17). For diazepam distribution volume increases almost linearly with age and thereby
also elimination half-life. But the average metabolic clearance remains
rather unchanged, although variability increases with age. As to sex differences, relatively little information is available for humans, but an interesting study recently revealed that the elimination half-life of chlordiazepoxide in females was almost twice as long as in males, whereas this
difference was almost threefold in females on oral contraceptives (19).
A similar study with nitrazepam did not reveal such substantial differences (20).

Cigarette smoking appears to induce oxidative drug metabolism rather
selectively and for instance theophylline clearance is almost twice as
high among smokers compared to non-smokers. Also diet is a factor of importance in relation to the rate of drug metabolism; high carbohydrate diet
tends to decrease the rate of metabolism whereas high protein tends to
increase it. Vegetarians seem to metabolize drugs at a lower rate.

As one would expect liver disease represents a situation during which
changes in the rate of metabolism will occur. It should be realized however,
that the term liver disease covers a great variety of pathological situations, which all may have different implications for drug metabolism. For
instance in extensive studies which were performed with the test compound
hexobarbital, it appeared that during acute hepatitis the average rate of
drug elimination was retarded, but large interpatient differences were
observed. These differences were even far greater among patients with
liver cirrhosis (Fig. 6). It is hard to predict to what extent the metabolism of a particular compound is affected in liver disease, because no
clear-cut correlations have been shown to exist between certain biochemical
or plasma enzyme values and for example metabolic clearance. Therefore
individualization of drug therapy according to clinical response is the
most appropriate manner by which to manage drugs in patients with liver
disease. With the use of induction agents it is to be expected that the
duration of residual effects is prolonged in patients with liver disease,

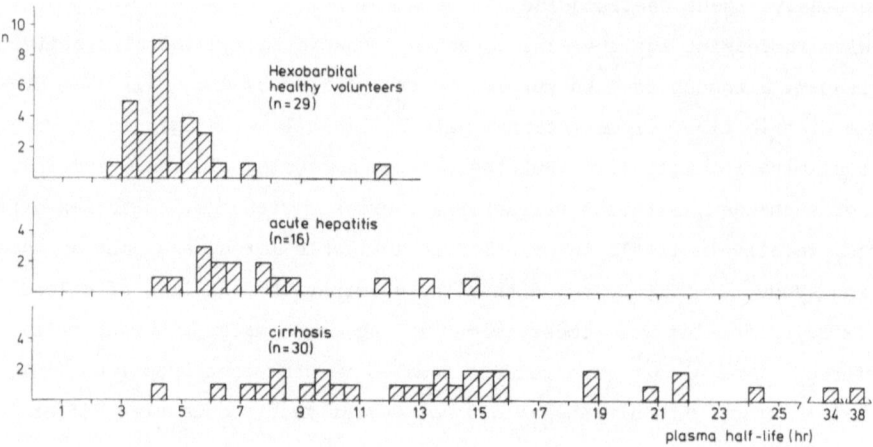

FIGURE 6. Frequency histogram (n = number of subjects) of plasma elimin-ation half-lives of hexobarbital in healthy volunteers, in patients with acute hepatitis and in patients with liver cirrhosis (16).

because this is mainly determined by the rate of metabolism. In thyroid disease generally the hypothyroid situation is associated with decreased and the hyperthyroid situation with increased rates of drug metabolism.

The problems of drug interactions in terms of induction or inhibition of drug metabolism is rather well documented. Barbiturates and most anti-epileptic agents are well-known inducers, but also the anti-tuberculous drug rifampicin is a potent compound in this regard. As a consequence dosage of concomitantly administered drugs has to be increased in order to obtain the same effect as before induction. It should be realized that in the course of multiple drug treatment, drug metabolizing activity may considerably change. Recently hexobarbital disposition was studied at different stages of intensive care treatment (21). At the beginning the average hexobarbital clearance was slightly reduced, whereas at later stages of treatment a substantial increase in metabolic clearance was observed (Fig. 7). Many factors play a role in such complicated clinical situations, but the multitude of drugs given to these patients is very

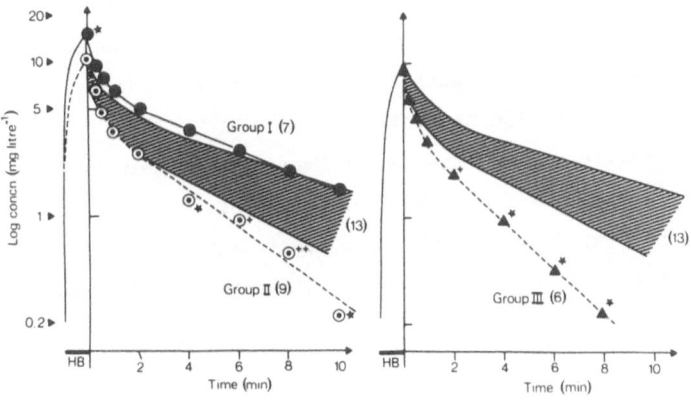

FIGURE 7. *Plasma concentration curves of hexobarbital following a 60-min zero-order i.v. infusion (7.3 mg/kg) into three groups of intensive-care patients: I, at the beginning of treatment; II, between 5 and 8 days after the beginning of treatment; III. between 13 and 29 days of treatment. The shaded area represents the range for healthy subjects. Data points indicate the mean values of the patients of the three groups (number of patients in brackets) (21).*

likely to be a major factor in the development of enzyme induction.

The hitherto discussed factors affecting the rate of drug metabolism are related to drug metabolizing activity at the enzymatic level (intrinsic metabolic clearance). It is important to note however that very rapidly metabolized drugs become dependent on hepatic blood flow as far as their total rate of elimination is concerned. This hold for the so-called high-clearance drugs like propranolol, lidocaine, methohexital, etomidate and many others. The duration of effect of such drugs is more sensitive to changes in hepatic blood flow than to changes in enzymatic activity. Decreased hepatic blood flow is associated with volume depletion, decreased cardiac output, heart failure, liver cirrhosis, circulatory collapse. Increased flow is caused by supine posture, food intake and some drugs (see for review: 22).

CONCLUSIONS

The pharmacokinetics of induction agents are to be considered as very relevant in relation to their onset and duration of anaesthetic action (drug distribution and redistribution) and duration of residual CNS depressant effects (drug elimination).

The pharmacokinetics of almost any drug varies considerably from one individual to the other, which means that often individualization of drug dosage is needed. It is important to consider the factors responsible for such variation, so that in clinical practice these can be taken into account.

REFERENCES

1. Rowland, M. and Tozer, T.N.: *Clinical Pharmacokinetics.*
    Lea & Febiger, Philadelphia, 1980.

2. Gibaldi, M. and Perrier, D.: *Pharmacokinetics.*
    Marcel Dekker Inc., New York, 1975.

3. Van Rossum, J.M.: *Farmacokinetiek – Cursus Postacademisch Onderwijs.*
    K.N.M.P., Den Haag, 1976.

4. Curry, S.H.: *Drug Disposition and Pharmacokinetics,* 3rd.,
    Blackwell Scientific Publications, Oxford, 1980.

5. Ghoneim, M.M. and Korttila, K.: Pharmacokinetics of intravenous anaesthetics: implications for clinical use. *Clinical Pharmacokinetics 2,* 344-372 (1977).

6. Duvaldestin, P.: Pharmacokinetics in intravenous anaesthetic practice. *Clinical Pharmacokinetics 6,* 61-82 (1981).

7. Sharma, R.P., Stowe, C.M. and Good, A.L.: Studies on the distribution and metabolism of thiopental in cattle, sheep, goats and swine. *The Journal of Pharmacology and Experimental Therapeutics 172,* 128-137 (1970).

8. Breimer, D.D.: Pharmacokinetics of methohexitone following intravenous infusion in humans. *British Journal of Anaesthesia 48,* 643-649 (1976).

9. Whitwam, J.G.: The pharmacology of brietal sodium (methohexitone sodium). *Anaesthesiologie und Wiederbelebung 57,* 1-19 (1972).

10. Breimer, D.D.: Clinical pharmacokinetics of hypnotics. *Clinical Pharmacokinetics 2,* 93-109 (1977).

11. Breimer, D.D., Jochemsen, R. and Von Albert, H.-H.: Pharmacokinetics of benzodiazepines: short-acting versus long-acting. *Arzneimittel-Forschung 30,* 875-881 (1980).

12. Schüttler, J., Stoeckel, H., Wilms, M., Schwilden, H. and Lauven, P.M.: Ein pharmakokinetisch begründetes Infusionsmodell für Etomidat zur Aufrechterhaltung von Steady State - Plasmaspiegeln. *Anaesthesist 29*, 662-666 (1980).

13. Dols, D.M., Burm, A.G., Middelburg, Y., Spierdijk, J. and Breimer, D.D.: Unpublished investigations.

14. De Wolff, F.A., Mattie, H. and Breimer, D.D. (eds). *Therapeutic Relevance of Drug Assays*. Boerhaave Series, Vol. 14, Leiden University Press, 1979.

15. Smith, S.E. and Rawlins, M.D. (eds). *Variability in Human Drug Response*. Butterworths, London, 1973.

16. Breimer, D.D. and Danhof, M.: Interindividual differences in pharmacokinetics and drug metabolism. In: *Towards Better Safety of Drugs and Pharmaceutical Products* (D.D. Breimer, ed.), Elsevier North-Holland Biomedical Press, Amsterdam, 1980, pp. 117-142.

17. Crooks, J. and Stevenson, I.H. (eds). *Drugs and the Elderly*. MacMillan Press, London, 1979.

18. Breimer, D.D., Zilly, W. and Richter, E.: Pharmacokinetics of hexobarbital in acute hepatitis and after apparent recovery. *Clinical Pharmacology and Therapeutics 18*, 433-440 (1975).

19. Roberts, R.K., Desmond, B.V., Wilkinson, G.R. and Schenker, S.: Disposition of chlordiazepoxide: sex differences and effects of oral contraceptives. *Clinical Pharmacology and Therapeutics 25*, 826-831 (1979).

20. Jochemsen, R., Van der Graaff, M., Boeijinga, J.K. and Breimer, D.D.: Influence of sex, menstrual cycle and oral contraception on the disposition of nitrazepam. *British Journal of Clinical Pharmacology*, in press (1981).

21. Rietbrock, I., Lazarus, G., Richter, E. and Breimer, D.D.: Hexobarbitone disposition at different stages of intensive care treatment. *British Journal of Anaesthesia 53*, 283-293 (1981).

22. Benet, L.Z. (ed). *The Effect of Disease States on Drug Pharmacokinetics*. American Pharmaceutical Association, Washington, 1976.

23. Dundee, J.W., Gamble, J.A.S. and Assaf, R.A.E.: Plasma-diazepam levels following intramuscular injection by nurses and doctors. *The Lancet 2*, 1461 (1974).

24. Ghoneim, M.M. and Van Hamme, M.J.: Pharmacokinetics of thiopentone. Effect of enflurane and nitrous oxide anaesthesia and surgery. *British Journal of Anaesthesia 50*, 1237-1241 (1978).

25. Wieber, J., Gugler, R., Hengstmann, J.H. and Dengler, H.J.: Pharmacokinetics of ketamine in man. *Anaestesist 24*, 260-263 (1975).

26. De Ruiter, G., Popescu, D.T., De Boer, A.G., Smeekens, J.B. and Breimer, D.D.: Pharmacokinetics of etomidate in surgical patients. *Archives internationales de Pharmacodynamie et de Thérapie 249,* 180-188 (1981).

27. Singlas, E.: Pharmacocinétique de flunitrazépam. *La Nouvelle Presse Médicale 8,* 2519-2523 (1979).

28. Smith, M.T., Eadie, M.J. and O'Rourke Brophy, T.: The pharmacokinetics of midazolam in man. *European Journal of Clinical Pharmacology 19,* 271-278 (1981).

MIDAZOLAM AS ANAESTHETIC INDUCTION AGENT

J.H. NAUTA, D.W. KOOPMAN, Joh. SPIERDIJK, T.H. STANLEY

Midazolam maleate (formerly designated RO 21-3981) (8-chloro-6(8-chloro-6 (2'-fluorophenyl)-1-methyl-4H miidazo- 1,5-a 1,4 benzodiazepine maleate) is a new benzodiazepine which is highly water soluble and stable in aqueous solutions[1].

Fig. 1

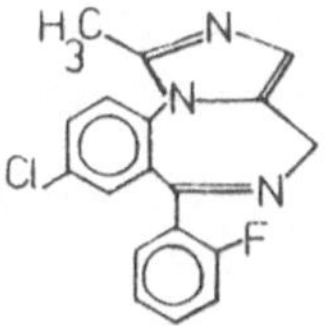

The water-solubility is the main difference between tne physical proper- ties of Midazolam and Diazepam[2]. Midazolam itself is highly lipofilic but its salts are watersoluble. Midazolam has all the well known pharmacologi- cal properties of the benzodiazepines (anxiolytic, sedative, anticonvul- sant, muscle relaxant actions, benign effects on other organ systems, low toxicity[2,3,4]. Midazolam is one and one-half times as potent as Diazepam and more rapid in action[2] (onset of induction 80 sec. vs. 94 sec. respec- tively).

Following rapid intravenous injection of Midazolam, plasma concentrations decrease to approximately 10% of peak blood levels within 1 hour. This appears to be related to a rapid redistribution[1,4,5]. The half-life in the β-fase, of the principle metabolite of midazolam (1-OH-Midazolam) ranges between about $1\frac{1}{2}$ and $2\frac{1}{2}$ hours[1,5].

Elimination of midazolam and its metabolites takes place principally in the liver and kidneys[1]. All metabolites of midazolam are pharmacologically inactive[1].

Used as an anaesthetic induction agent, Midazolam maleate is about 20 times as potent as thiopental. Thus 0.15 mg/kg of midazolam is equivalent to 3 mg/kg thiopental[4]. Induction with thiopental is about twice as fast as with Midazolam. An induction with 0.15-0.2 mg/kg of Midazolam (which appear to be doses required for induction) takes about 90 seconds in seco-barbital sedated patients[2,3,6,7]. However a dose of 0.15 mg/kg of the drug appears to be inadequate to induce anaesthesia in unpremedicated young subjects[2,6].

A combination of fentanyl with Midazolam gives a more rapid induction[7]. At equivalent sleep doses Midazolam is less likely to cause apnea than thiopental[4,7]. Venous irritation following Midazolam is infrequent and when it occurs is very mild. Some patients do experience a slight burning feeling on injection of midazolam[2,4,8,6]. Phlebitis, as is often reported after diazepam has not been observed after midazolam[2,4,6,8,9,7].

Cardiovascular parameters remain stable during induction with midazolam, what changes that do occur seem to be confined to arterial blood pressure which tends to decrease and heart rate which tends to raise [2,3,5,6,8]. The cardiovascular stability of Midazolam is about the same as that of Diazepam, even in cardiac patients[2,9].

The cardiovascular response to intubation, as with many other induction agents,is eliminated by Midazolam[3,11]. Midazolam induction appears to reduce halothane requirements during operation[12].

Recovery after Midazolam is slower than recovery after thiopental. After an induction dose of 0.15 mg/kg patients respond to commands in about 4-8 minutes. In about 45 minutes patients are fully conscious[4,5,7]. Amnesia following Midazolam lasts approximately one to two hours but may be longer[7]. No rebound sedation, as with diazepam, is seen[7]. Post-operative nausea and vomiting is less than after pentothal[7]. All of this suggests that the properties of Midazolam as an anaesthetic induction agent are not greatly different than the properties of the well known anaesthetic induction agent etomidate. Therefore the objective of this study was to evaluate Midazolam as anaesthetic induction agent in comparison with etomidate.

Methods

The experimental subjects included 40 patients without a history of cardiac, pulmonary or renal disease, about to undergo general surgical operations lasting from 30 minutes to 3 hours. The patients were taking no pre-operative medications. The ages ranged from 18 years to 70 years.

Two hours before the operation patients received a dose of 100 mg of seco-barbital orally. Half an hour before operation the patients received an intramuscular dose of $\frac{1}{2}$ mg of atropine.

Upon arrival in the operating room an intravenous infusion was established in a hand vein and continuous recording of bipolar lead II of the electro-cardiogram was started.

The following parameters were measured: systolic and diastolic blood pressures, and heart rate.

After preparatory measurements the patients were given a pre-curarizing dose of pancuronium of 1.25 mg/50 kg intravenously and allowed to breathe oxygen. Three minutes after pancuronium a rapid infusion of either etomidate (0.3 mg/kg) or Midazolam (0.2 mg/kg) was started. Administration of the drugs was randomized. The total dose of both drugs was administered in 30 seconds. During infusion the patients were commanded to take a deep breath every 5-10 seconds. Failure to respond to this command and loss of palpebral re-flexes were equated with unconsciousness. When unconscious, the patients were intubated following an intravenous dose of 1 mg/kg body-weight of succinylcholine.

One minute after intubation the patients received halothane and nitrous oxide in oxygen as the only anaesthetics for the rest of the operation. All patients were paralysed with pancuronium during operation. Cardiovascular dynamics were recorded before pancuronium administration, at the moment of unconsciousness, one minute after succinylcholine and one and four minutes after endotracheal intubation. Other variables evaluated during induction and intubation included pain on injection, the presence of arrhythmias, muscle movements and the time to unconsciousness.

During operation the dose of halothane required was recorded. At the end of the operation patients were extubated after reversal of the neuromus-cular blockade and transported to the recovery room for a stay of 120-180 minutes. In the recovery room the incidence of vomiting, the need for anal-gesics and the recovery time were recorded. The recovery time was the time the patients needed to become well oriented to time, place and person.

All patients were interviewed 24-48 hours postoperatively. Questions were specifically directed at determining the last and the first thing re-membered before and after induction of anaesthesia, the incidence of vomiting, other negative features of the recovery period and whether the patients remembered any aspect of the procedure after induction.

Results

The ages, weights, systolic and diastolic blood pressures and the heart rates of the two groups were similar. Seven patients of the etomidate group complained about pain on injection of the drug while, even when specifically asked, none of the patients of the Midazolam group experienced any pain on injection.

Systolic blood pressures remained very stable after injection of both drugs.

Table I
SBP (torr)

	Control	Unconscious	SDC	Intubate	Anesth.
Etomidate	134	135	138	162^X	129
Midazolam	139	144	138	168^X	140

$^X P < 01$, students paired t-test when compared to control values.

Heart rate remained stable after etomidate injection. A slight increase in heart rate was seen after Midazolam injection.

Table II
HR (beats/min)

	Control	Unconscious	SDC	Intubate	Anesth.
Etomidate	81	84	91	105^+	90
Midazolam	80	94^X	99^X	109^+	103

$^X P < 05$, $^+ P < 01$, students paired t-test when compared to control values.

Following laryngoscopy and intubation systolic blood pressures increased significantly (21%), above control values in both groups (table I).

The increase in heart rate following intubation was in the Midazolam group of patients higher (36%) than in the etomidate group of patients (30%) but this difference was not significant (table II).

Induction with Midazolam averaged 116 seconds (45-390 sec.). Induction with etomidate averaged 62 seconds. The induction dose of Midazolam varied over a wide range (0.18-0.4 mg/kg) with a mean value of 0.24 $\pm$ 0.07 mg/kg.

Mean dose of etomidate was 0.30 ± 0.01 mg/kg.

In both groups muscle movements of any kind during induction and intubation occurred in about 45% of patients. Muscle movements after Midazolam occurred mostly during intubation in contrast to the muscle movements of etomidate which occurred mostly after injection.

One patient in each group experienced premature ventricular contractions during induction and intubation. These arrhythmias were transient and did not need therapeutic measures. Halothane intraoperative requirement were about the same in both groups of patients, ranging from 0.6% to 0.9%.

Table III

	Sleep time seconds	Muscle move (%)	Injection pain (%)	Haloth.range (%)
Etomidate	62	45	35	0,7-0,9
Midazolam	116	45	0	0,6-0,9

Postoperatively the patients who received Midazolam took about 40 minutes to recover consciousness while patients who received etomidate needed 30 minutes. In the early postoperative period 75% of the patients who received etomidate needed analgesics versus 45% of patients who received Midazolam.

The patients who received etomidate experienced significantly more vomiting (55%) than the patients who received Midazolam (15%).

	Vomiting	% Analgetics	Time (min) Analg.
Etomidate	55%	75	40
Midazolam	15%	45	52

The last thing all the patients remembered before unconsciousness was the mask was being placed on their face.

Postoperatively only one patient of the etomidate group remembered being awake in the operating room. All other patients woke up in the recovery room.

Discussion

The results of this study indicate that the new potent water soluble benzodiazepine, midazolam, is an anaesthetic induction agent, which is in many respects comparable to etomidate. Until laryngoscopy and intubation, systolic blood pressure remain as stable as with etomidate.

The slight increase in heart rate after Midazolam is the only difference
in cardiovascular performance of both drugs. Neither Midazolam nor Etomidate
eliminate the cardiovascular responses of laryngoscopy and intubation which
are also seen with many other induction agents[11]. This cardiovascular
stimulation (hypertension and tachycardia) is of about the same magnitude
with both drugs. Induction with Midazolam lasts twice as long as induction
with etomidate. In our study the induction dose of midazolam varied a great
deal. We think, this was due to the light preoperative sedation. In contrast to etomidate not one of our patients experienced pain on injection.
The muscle movements seen with midazolam occurred mostly during laryngoscopy and intubation. In our opinion those muscle movements were due to
incomplete muscle relaxation and as such not unlike muscle movements seen
with thiopentone. In contrast muscle movements following etomidate occurred
mostly after injection (myolonic movements).

Our results indicate that midazolam has a somewhat longer duration of
action than etomidate. Etomidate patients became conscious faster and
needed more analgesics early postoperatively than patients in the midazolam group. This could be the reason for the high incidence of vomiting
which occurred in the etomidate group.

In conclusion: Midazolam is a potent, pain-free anaesthetic induction
agent with the same cardiovascular benignity as etomidate.

Onset of action with midazolam takes twice as much time as the onset of
action of etomidate in lightly sedated patients. Recovery after midazolam
seems to take somewhat more time than recovery after etomidate. Patients
who received midazolam needed less analgesics in the early post-operative
period and vomited less than patients who received etomidate. Muscle
movements after midazolam occurred mostly during laryngoscopy and intubation and were possibly due to an incomplete paralysis.

References

1. Amrein, R., Cano, J.P., Eckert, M.: Metabolismus und Pharmakokinetisches Verhalten von Midazolam.
   Proceedings Assemblée annuelle de la société Suisse d'Anaesthésiologie et de Réanimation, Midazolam Symposium Genève 26-28 June 1980.

2. Reves, J.G., Corssen, G., Holcomb, C.: Comparison of two benzodiazepines for Anaesthesis induction: Midazolam and Diazepam.
   Canad. An. Soc. J. 25, no.3, 211-214 (1978).

3. Schwander, D., Sansano, C.: Cardiovascular changes during intubation with Midazolam as anaesthetic induction agent.
   Proceedings Assemblée annuelle de la Société Suisse d'Anaesthésiologie et de Réanimation, Midazolam Symposium Genève 26-28 June 1980.

4. Sarnquist, F.H., Mathers, W.D., Brock-Utne, J., Carr, B., Canup, C., Brown, C.R.: A Bioassay of a water-soluble benzodiazepine against sodium Thiopental.
   Anesthesiology 52: 149-153, 1980.

5. Brown, C.R., Sarnquist, F.H., Canup, A.C., Pedley, T.A.: Clinical electroencephalographic, and pharmacokinetic studies of a water-soluble benzodiazepine, Midazolam maleate.
   Anesthesiology 50: 467-470, 1979.

6. Forster, A., Gardaz, J.P., Suter, P.M., Gemperle, M.: I.V. Midazolam as an induction agent for anaesthesia: A study in volunteers.
   Br. J. Anaesth. 52: 907, 1980.

7. Fragen, R.J., Caldwell, N.: Awakening characteristics following induction with midalolam for short surgical procedures.
   Proceedings Assemblée annuelle de la Société Suisse d'Anaesthésiologie et de Réanimation, Midazolam Symposium Genève 26-28 June 1980.

8. Fragen, R.J., Gahl, F., Caldwell, N.: A water soluble benzodiazepine, RO 21-3981, for induction of anaesthesia.
   Anesthesiol. 49: 41-43, 1978.

9. Greenblatt, D.J., Shader, R.I.: Benzodiazepines in clinical practice, p. 203, Raven Press, New York, 1974.

10. Fragen, R.J., Meyers, S.N., Barresi, V., Caldwell, N.J.: Hemodynamic effects of Midazolam in cardiac patients.
    Anesthesiol. 51, no. 3, 103, Sept. 1979.

11. Popescu, D.T.: Clinical experience with etomidate.
    In: Anaesthesia and Pharmacology, Boerhaave series 12, p. 152,
    Leiden. University Press, 1976.
12. Melvin, M.A., Johnson, B.H., Quasha, A.L., Eger II, E.I.: Induction
    of anesthesia with Midazolam decreases halothane MAC in man.
    Anesthesiol. 53, no. 3, 10, Sept. 1980.

DIPRIVAN

L. VERSICHELEN, G. ROLLY and N.A. ZUBAIR

Anaesthetic activity has been discovered in a series of hindered phenolic compounds which exist as oils at room temperature. These coumpounds can be given I.V. in aquous solution with a solubilizing agent. Of the compóunds examined only I.C.I. 35868 (Diprivan) was found to have a desirable anaesthetic profile in animals. Diprivan or 2,6-diisopropylphenol has a very simple chemical structure (fig. 1).

Chemically it is unrelated to any of the currently used barbiturate, eugenol or steroid anaesthetic agents. Despite the low solubility in water, an aquous solution can be prepared using Cremophor E.L., although this in itself induces some problems.

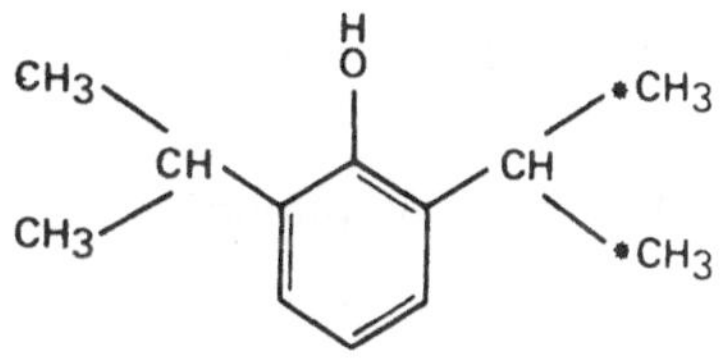

Figure 1. DIPRIVAN

In animals it has been shown that Diprivan rapidly produces anaesthesia of short duration (1). Pharmacokinetic studies demonstrated that it has an extremely short distribution half-life (1-6 minutes) and that the terminal elimination phase is also short (16-55 minutes) (2). The pharmacologic prophile is such that Diprivan is apparently suitable *both* for induction and for maintenance of anaesthesia. Rapid metabolic breakdown in rabbits prevented the attainment of anaesthetic blood concentrations after I.M. administration (1).

In mice it has been shown that after a faster rate of
I.V. injection, a much smaller dose of Diprivan was required for the same anaesthetic effect. EEG changes produced
by Diprivan in the rat indicate a profound, but rapidly
reversed depression of cerebral activity, suggesting that
the dose response curve for this effect seems steeper with
Diprivan than with barbiturates, with the result that little
hypnosis is likely as bloodconcentration decreases to less
than that required to produce unconsciousness. No vein damage occurred after I.V. injection in animals, nor necro-
sis following perivascular injection.

The anaesthetic activity has been reported in human volunteers and in patients in 1977 (3). In those initial studies made during epidural anaesthesia, sleep was induced
with an I.V. dose of 0.75-1 mg/kg. Further studies have
shown that the onset of sleep is rapid and smooth and without muscle movement. Mild pain occurs in the hand or arm
on injection, and is one of the major drawbacks of this
drug.

Diisopropylphenol or Diprivan is provided as a 1 % solution, in 16 % Cremophor E.L. and is presented in amp. of
10 ml. The injection through an ordinary needle is fairly
easy, but when a high injection speed is wanted smaller
needles are less easy.

Till up now, diisopropylphenol has been used in several
trials in the U.K. and in Belgium, whereby the effectiveness as induction agent was assessed (4), and later on in
studies for maintenance with repetitive doses or by constant
infusion. Authorisation has been given up till now to use
the drug in healthy patients of ASA Class I and II.

In our department, we had experience with the use of
diisopropylphenol as induction agent, in 2 groups of ASA I
patients, a first group of 39 patients and a second one of
32 patients.

The first study was in fact a dose finding and general
evaluation study, in wich Diprivan was injected in 9 male
and 30 female patients, aged 17-65 years, scheduled to un-

dergo minor surgical procedures (5). In all patients Diprivan was injected I.V. over 30 seconds, without premedication,
into a small vein of the dorsus of the hand, or into a larger forearm vein. The first 6 patients were given 1.0 mg/kg,
the next 22 1.5 mg/kg, the final 11 2.0 mg/kg. Anaesthesia was successfully induced only in 50 % of the patients
at 1.0 mg/kg dose, 81 % at a 1.5 mg/kg dose and 100 % at a
2.0 mg/kg dose. The sleep induction times were respectively
53 ± 13, 50 ± 4 and 40 ± 4 seconds (Mean + SEM) after start
of injection. The major drawback was the occurrence of pain
at the injection site in 23 % of patients, but there were no
signs of venous damage postoperatively.

A small, transient fall in bloodpressure and in the 2.0
mg/kg group an increase in heartrate were seen (fig. 2).

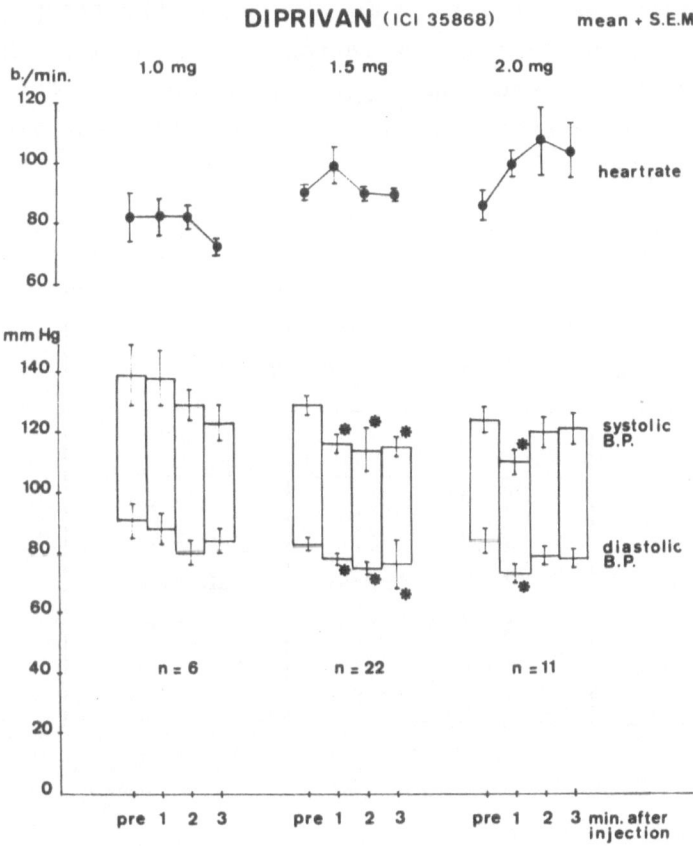

Figure 2. Cardiovascular parameters after Diprivan injection (5).

Respiratory depression was seen immediately after induction;
transient apnoea occurred in 27 % of patients given 1.5 mg/
kg and 55 % given 2.0 mg/kg. Three minutes after induction
of anaesthesia, when assessments were complete 23 patients
were given a further dose of another induction agent, as
they were beginning to awaken.

A dose of 1.5 mg/kg was considered appropriate for further examination in a second study, in which the usefulness
of premedication and the influence of speed of injection
were assessed (6). Diprivan was always injected in a very
fast running I.V. drip, at an injection speed of 10 or 20
seconds, and after premedication with 0.1 mg fentanyl (F)
or not (S); 32 ASA I female patients, scheduled for minor
gynaecological surgery, were assigned by randomisation to
the 4 equal subgroups (F10, F20, S10, S20). The sleep induction times showed that the faster injection rate, the
quicker induction speed and especially if compared to the
first group, whereby the influence of injection rate is
evident (Table 1).

Table 1.

Diprivan 1 % Induction time	1.5 mg/kg (seconds)	
	Mean + SEM	Range
F 10	39.4 $\pm$ 8.9	10 - 85
F 20	45.4 $\pm$ 2.4	40 - 60
S 10	36.6 $\pm$ 4.7	20 - 55
S 20	44.4 $\pm$ 3.1	29 - 60
S 30	50.0 $\pm$ 4.0	30 - 90

Sleep was successfully induced in all patients. The response to a painful stimulus applied 1 minute after injection,
showed that still 19 patients had slight movement and 10
gross movement, whereby more movement in the non premedicated group than in the other.

After injection, systolic and diastolic bloodpressures
decreased, significantly in 3 groups (fig. 3). Heartrate
decreased in all groups, but not significantly.

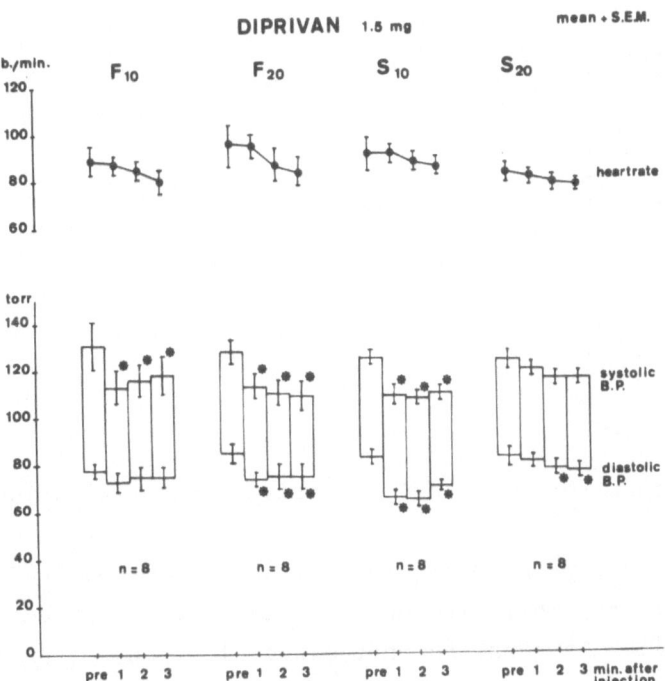

Fig. 3. Cardiovascular parameters after Diprivan injection (6).

Respiratory rate decreased significantly at 1 minute after start of injection (fig. 4). In the F 10 groups, we had
one patient developping a very pronounced tachypnoea, that
might will have been a discrete intolerance reaction to the
Cremophor solubiliser, although none of our patients had received this drug before. Apnoea of at least 15 seconds was
present in 20 patients, with a mean apnoea time of 30 - 35
seconds.

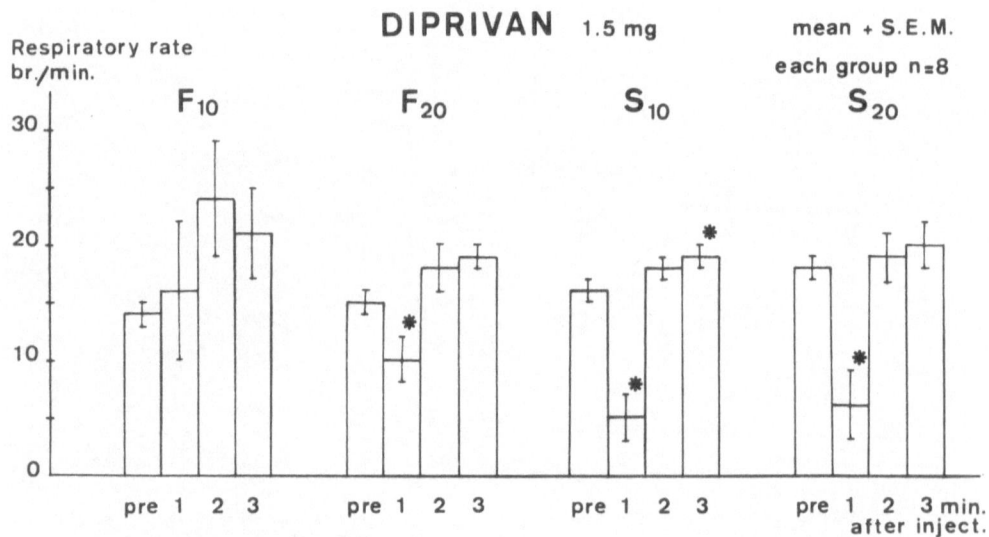

Figure 4. Respiratory rate after Diprivan injection (6).

In this study, pain during injection was present in 4
patients (12.5 %), while in the first trial it occurred in
23 % of patients, suggesting that direct I.V. injection is
more discomforting. Although venous irritation is not a
major problem, it has to be improved for the future and an
alternative solubilising agent probably has to be looked
for. Other side effects as vomiting and nausea were low.

In other studies, Diprivan was used for maintenance of inconsciousness during locoregional blocks, or for providing total intravenous anaesthesia. Dose ranges of 68 µg/kg/min. to 200 µg/kg/min. are mentioned (7). These studies clearly show no accumulation of the drug in the body (8).

It is at this moment too early to make a definite statement on the future place of Diprivan in anaesthesia. The quick onset of action and minor side effects are useful characteristics; the transient apnoe is not of major concern. The absence of cumulation is certainly a plus for the maintenance dose regime. The incidence of pain on injection is nevertheless at the present formulation a drawback, but can be minimised by injection in fastrunning infusions.

REFERENCES

1. Glen J.B. 1980. Animal studies of the anaesthetic activity of ICI 35868. Brit.J.Anaesth., 52, 731-743.
2. Adam H.K., Glen J.B., Hoyle P.A. 1980. Pharmacokinetics in laboratory animals of ICI 35868, a new I.V. anaesthetic agent. Brit.J.Anaesth., 52, 743-747.
3. Kay B., Rolly G. 1977. ICI 35868, a new intravenous induction agent. Acta Anaesth. Belg., 28, 303-317.
4. Rogers K.M., Dewar K.M.S., McCublin T.D., Spence A.A.1980. Preliminary experience with ICI 35868 as an I.V. induction agent : comparison with Althesin.
Brit.J.Anaesth., 52, 807-811.
5. Rolly G., Versichelen L., Zubair N.A. 1980. Use of ICI 35868 as an anaesthetic induction agent. Acta Anaesth. Belg., 31, 241-244.
6. Rolly G., Versichelen L., Zubair N.A. 1981. Effects of premedication and speed of injection on induction of anaesthesia with ICI 35868 (DiprivanR). To be published in the Proceedings of the European Academy of Anaesthesiology.
7. Savege T. 1981. Preliminary report on the use of Diprivan for total intravenous anaesthesia. Investigators Meeting at I.C.I., March 1981.
8. Kay B. 1981. Diprivan (ICI 35868), a new intravenous induction agent. Proceedings World Congress of Anesthesiology, International Congress Series 538, Excerpta Medica, 728-732.

ALFENTANYL: A NEW NARCOTIC ANAESTHETIC INDUCTION AGENT

J.H. NAUTA, S. DE LANGE, D.W. KOOPMAN, J.W. VAN KLEEF, JOH. SPIERDIJK,
Th.H. STANLEY

Since it's introduction in the early 1960's fentanyl has acquired a good reputa-
tion as narcotic analgesic in anaesthesia. The drug meets most of the requirements for an analgesic in anaesthesia. For this reason fentanyl has become the
predecessor of a series of highly potent narcotic analgesics. One of the recent
ly synthesized derivatives is alfentanyl (R 39 209).

Fig. 1

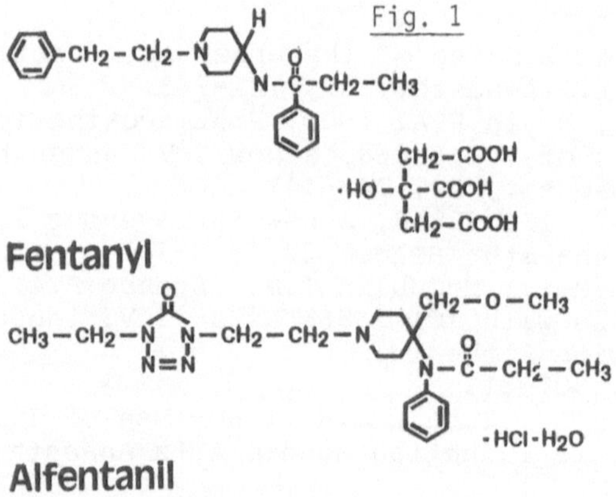

Fentanyl

Alfentanil

Animal tests have shown alfentanyl to have a duration of action of 1/3 of fentanyl. The onset of action of alfentanyl is very rapid (one circulation time if
given as a bolus)* The duration of action of a single dose is less than five
minutes.
The potency of alfentanyl is 1/3 of the potency of fentanyl. The margin of
safety between toxic and effective dose is very high (about 1000). [1,2]
Furthermore alfentanyl has an apparent benignity on circulatory dynamics. All
this suggests that alfentanyl might be useful as an anaesthetic induction agent
[1,2] The objective of this investigation was to evaluate alfentanyl as an
anaesthetic induction agent in patients with and without significant cardiovas-

*de Castro, J., (Personal communication)

cular disease.

Methods

The experimental subjects included 20 patients without a history of cardiac, pulmonary or renal disease about to undergo general surgical operations group I. Group II consisted of 9 patients with severe mitral valvular disease (stenosis and/or insufficiency) about to undergo mitral valvular replacement. Group III consisted of 13 patients with coronary artery disease about to undergo coronary artery bypass grafting operations. Patients in group I were taking no pre-operative medications while all but one of those in group II were taking digoxin and one or more of a variety of diuretics. All patients in group III were taking propranolol and ten nitroglycerin or another vasodilator as well.

Patients in group I were premedicated with atropine while those in group II and III were given lorazepam and atropine. Patients taking propranolol received their usual dose of oral propranolol at the time of the premedication. Upon arrival in the operating room a catheter was placed in a hand vein and the continuous recording of bipolar lead II of the electrocardiogram was started. The following parameters were measured: systolic and diastolic bloodpressure, heart rate and respiratory rate in patients of group I, radial arterial pressures, mean right arterial pressure, pulmonary arterial pressure and cardiac output in patients in group II and III.

Following preparatory procedures and a 10 minute stabilization period, control cardiovascular dynamics were recorded and the patients given oxygen to breathe. Two minutes later pancuronium (1.5 mg/70 kg) was administered intravenously. Three minutes after pancuronium, alfentanyl was administered at 3.5 mg/minute intravenously. During infusion of alfentanyl, patients were commanded to open their eyes and take a deep breath every 5-10 seconds. Failure to respond to three consecutive commands was equated with unconsciousness.

When unconscious, the patients were intubated following succinylcholine. One minute after intubation patients in group I received halothane and nitrous oxide in oxygen as the only other anaesthetics for the remainder of the operatio while patients in group II and III received additional alfentanyl. All patients were paralyzed with pancuronium during operation. Cardiovascular dynamics were recorded before and three minutes after pancuronium administration, at the moment of unconsciousness, one minute after succinylcholine and one and four minutes after endotracheal intubation. Other variables evaluated during induction included: pain with alfentanyl injection; the presence of arrhythmias; muscle

movements; chest wall rigidity according to a 3 point scale: the time to unconsciousness and the dose of alfentanyl needed for unconsciousness. At the end
of the operation the patients in group I were extubated after reversal of the
neuromuscular blockade if their respiration was adequate (f 12/min. TV 7 ml/kg).
The somnolence score was determined via the method of Bidwai.[3] On entrance to
the recovery room, 5 and 15 minutes later and every 15 minutes thereafter for
three hours.

Patients in group II and III were all electively mechanically ventilated until
the morning after surgery. During the first eight post-operative hours these
patients were evaluated for return of consciousness every 15 minutes and, once
conscious, the ability to sustain adequate spontaneous respiration every 30
minutes.

Patients were considered conscious when they could give correct affirmative or
negative responses to three consecutive questions. Patients in group II and III
were considered ready for extubation when they had   stable cardiovascular
dynamics for two hours and when they could sustain adequate spontaneous respiration.

All patients were interviewed 24-48 hours post-operatively. Questions were
specifically directed at determining the last and the first things remembered
before and after induction of anaesthesia, the incidence of vomiting, other
negative features of the recovery period and whether the patients remembered
any aspect of the procedure after alfentanyl.

Results

The ages, weights and pre-operative diastolic bloodpressures of the three
groups were similar. Group I had a significantly higher pre-operative systolic
arterial bloodpressure than groups II and III and significantly higher pre-
operative heart rate than group III.

Patients in group I needed 119 μg of alfentanyl for induction, while those in group II and III needed 41 and 50 μg/kg respectively.

Table 1

PRE-OPERATIVE DATA (MEAN $\pm$ SD)

	Age (years)	Weight (kg)	Pre-anaesthetic heart rate (beats/min)	Pre-anaesthetic blood pressure Systolic (torr)	Diastolic (torr)
Group I	42 $\pm$10	72 $\pm$10	85 $\pm$ 9	143 $\pm$ 10	70 $\pm$ 9
Group II	48 $\pm$11	63 $\pm$ 9	78 $\pm$ 8	128* $\pm$ 11	68 $\pm$ 7
Group III	51 $\pm$ 9	73 $\pm$ 8	72* $\pm$ 9	130* $\pm$ 9	64 $\pm$ 9

* $P < .05$, students unpaired t-test, when compared to group 1 values at the same

No patient in either group experienced pain upon intravenous injection of al-fentanyl and only one patient (group I) experienced an arrhythmia lasting 45 seconds during endotracheal intubation. Some muscle movements (usually during laryngoscopy) occurred in five patients in group 1 but in no other patient in either group.

Table 2

TABLE OF ALFENTANYL REQUIRED FOR UNCONSCIOUSNESS
AND OPERATION AND ANAESTHETIC INDUCTION TIME
(Mean $\pm$ SD)

	Alfentanyl (ug/kg)		Induction time
	Unconscious	Operation	(seconds)
Group I	119 $\pm$ 20	119 $\pm$ 20	134 $\pm$ 28
Group II	41* $\pm$ 9	746 $\pm$ 81	47* $\pm$ 19
Group III	50*+ $\pm$ 10	1356+ $\pm$ 120	75* ## $\pm$ 22

* P $<$.01, Chi-Square test when compared to Group I values at
the same time

P $<$.05, + P $<$.01, Chi-Square test when compared to group II
values at the same time

Table 3

ANAESTHETIC INDUCTION DATA (% OF PATIENTS)

	Pain on injection	Muscle movements	Chest Wall Rigidity			Arrhythmias
			Mild	Severe	Total	
Group I	0	25	30	20	50	5
Group II	0	0	22	0	22*	0
Group III	0	0	23	8	31*	0

* P $<$.025, Chi-Square test when compared to group I values

Fifty percent of the patients in group I experienced some form of chest wall rigidity during induction.

The incidence of chest wall rigidity was significantly less in groups II and III, 22 and 31 percent respectively. Rigidity was severe enough to totally inhibit positive pressure ventilation before succinylcholine in five patients (four patients in group I and one in group III).

With the exception of systolic arterial bloodpressure which was slightly increased following pancuronium and slightly decreased at the moment at which unconsciousness first occurred, no other cardiovascular variable was significantly changed at any time during the study period in patients in groups II and III.

Table 4

CARDIOVASCULAR RESPONSES DURING ANAESTHETIC INDUCTION
WITH ALFENTANYL (Mean $\pm$ SD)

		Control	Pancuronium	Unconscious	Succinylcholine	Intubation 1 min.	Intubation 4 min.
Heart rate	I	85 ± 9	$96\pm9^+$	$103\pm10^+$	$105\pm11^+$	$109\pm11^+$	86 ± 9
(beats/min)	II	78 ± 8	$80\pm7^*$	$70\pm7^*$	$76\pm7^*$	$72\pm8^*$	$71\pm7^*$
	III	$72\pm9^*$	$76\pm7^*$	$67\pm6^*$	$69\pm7^*$	$71\pm8^*$	$68\pm8^*$
Systolic blood	I	143 ± 10	$153\pm9^+$	$153\pm10^+$	$154\pm9^+$	$158\pm9^+$	137 ± 10
Pressure (torr)	II	$128\pm11^*$	$136\pm8^{*+}$	$117\pm9^{*+}$	$123\pm8^*$	$124\pm7^*$	$122\pm8^*$
	III	$130\pm9^*$	$137\pm9^{*+}$	$118\pm12^{*+}$	$121\pm11^*$	$126\pm11^*$	123 ± 10
Diastolic blood	I	70 ± 9	72 ± 8	69 ± 9	71 ± 8	73 ± 8	64 ± 7
Pressure (torr)	II	68 ± 7	72 ± 7	60 ± 10	63 ± 9	66 ± 8	65 ± 7
	III	64 ± 9	66 ± 8	61 ± 9	62 ± 7	64 ± 7	61 ± 8
Mean right arterial	II	6 ± 2	6 ± 2	8 ± 3	8 ± 2	5 ± 2	6 ± 2
Pressure (torr)	III	8 ± 2	8 ± 2	9 ± 2	8 ± 2	9 ± 2	9 ± 2
Mean pulmonary artery	II	17 ± 2	19 ± 2	16 ± 3	18 ± 2	18 ± 2	15 ± 2
Pressure (torr)	III	17 ± 2	17 ± 2	19 ± 3	19 ± 2	17 ± 2	16 ± 2
Cardiac output	II	4.6 ± 0.5	5.2 ± 0.7	4.2 ± 0.7	4.4 ± 0.7	18 ± 2	4.2 ± 0.5
(l/min)	III	6.0 ± 0.7	5.1 ± 0.8	5.8 ± 0.9	5.6 ± 0.8	17 ± 2	5.5 ± 0.7

+ $P < .05$, paired t-test when compared to control values

* $P < .05$, analysis of variance when compared to Group I values

In contrast, patients in group I experienced significant increases in heart rat
and systolic arterial bloodpressure following pancuronium which were maintained
until four minutes following intubation (when anaesthesia was being maintained
with halothane and nitrous oxide).

All patients in group 1 could be extubated at the end of the operation and
all were responding to verbal command upon entrance to the recoevery room.

All patients in group I were considered ready for discharge from the recovery
room within 30 minutes of arriving.

Retching and/or vomiting occurred in four patients in group I during the three
hour mandatory recovery room stay but did not re-occur thereafter during the
following 24 hours. None of the other patients in any of the groups experienced nausea, retching or vomiting at any time during the first 24 post-
operative hours.

With the exception of one patient (in group III) all patients in groups II and
III were conscious within three hours of the end of the operation. Mean times
for fulfiliment of the criteria for endotracheal extubation in groups II and
III were 6.3 and 4.1 hours respectively. Only one patient in each group II and
II could not have been extubated, according to our criteria for extubation, by
the end of the eight post-operative hour.

Table 5

RECOVERY TIMES ON 22 PATIENTS ANAESTHETIZED
WITH ALFENTANYL FOR MITRAL VALVULAR AND CABG OPERATIONS
(Mean $\pm$ SD)

	Consciousness (hrs)	Ready for + Extubation (hrs)	Patients not ready for extubation 8 hours post-operatively (%)
Group II	13 $\pm$ 0.6	6.3 $\pm$ 1.2	11
Group III	1.4 $\pm$ 0.8	4.1* $\pm$ 1.5	8

* P < .05, unpaired t-test when compared to group II values at the same time

+ Data in this column are only from patients who were considered ready for
  endotracheal extubation before the 9th post-operative hour

When interviewed post-operatively, all patients in group I related that the last thing they remembered was a mask being placed on their face and the first thing after anaesthesia, their presence in the operating or recovery room. Forty-one percent of group II and III patients never remembered ever coming to the operating room and of the remainder, only two patients remembered a face mask being applied. Patients in groups II and III first memory after operation was usually the appearance of one of their family members with them in the intensive care unit 6-20 hours post-operatively. No patient in the study remembered laryngoscopy, endotracheal intubation or any aspect of the operative procedure. However, one patient in group I did recall being stiff just before unconsciousness and it frightened her.

Discussion

The results of this study indicate that the new ultra-short acting synthetic narcotic alfentanyl can be used as an anaesthetic induction agent prior to intubation and anaesthesia. Induction with alfentanyl is smooth and reasonably fast especially in patients who are well sedated as were patients in groups II and III. These patients became unconscious within one minute and a half after alfentanyl.

Unsedated patients (group I) took somewhat longer for induction but were unconscious. Not one of our patients experienced pain on injection. The hypnotic action of alfentanyl appears to be reasonably good, only one patient from Group I remebered being stiff just before she became unconscious.

In five patients of group I we saw some muscle movement during laryngoscopy, not one of these occurred during or shortly after injection.

Cardiovascular parameters remained very stable during induction and intubation in all patients. This is a very promising sign, for cardiovascular instability during induction and intubation is quite common with most available induction agents.[4] Only one patient (group I had a arrhythmia (PVS) and this occurred during extubation.

A dose of 1.5 mg/70 kg of pancuronium before induction was not enough to abolish alfentanyl induced chest wall rigidity in all patients. This chest wall rigidity can be a serious problem. However, it appears to be reduced by premedication with lorazepam and is eliminated by succinylcholine.

No patient experienced bradycardia after alfentanyl, as has been seen by other investigators[5]. This was probably due to the pancuronium dose before the induction as were the elevated heart rate and systolic bloodpressure seen in group I.

The data suggest that the duration of respiratory depression due to alfentanyl is short. Not one of the patients in group I needed a narcotic antagonist before extubation at the end of the operation.

All patients in group I were alert and able to converse within 15 minutes of entry into the recovery room. Six patients of this group needed analgesics and four of those six patients experienced nausea and/or vomiting afterwards. It is difficult to say if this nausea and vomiting was due to the given analgesics or to the action of alfentanyl.

In conclusion: Alfentanyl is a rapid-acting, pain-free, narcotic anesthetic induction agent which produced hypnosis, little alteration in cardiovascular dynamics and a minimum of muscle movements.

The duration of respiratory depression with alfentanyl appears to be short. While chest wall rigidity can be a problem with alfentanyl anesthetic induction, it can be reduced with a lorazepam premedication (as can cardiovascular stimulation from pancuronium and intubation) and eliminated with succinylcholine.

References

1. de Castro, J., Van de Water, A., Wouters, L., et al.: A comparative study of cardiovascular, neurological and metabolic side-effects of eight narcotics in dogs. Acta Anaesthesiolog. Belg. 30: 5-99, 1979.

2. de Castro, J.: Practical application and limitations of analgesic anaesthesia. Acta Anaesthesiolog. Belg. 27: 107-128, 1976.

3. Bidwai, A.V., Cornelius, L.R., Stanley, T.H.: Reversal of Innovarinduced post anaesthetic somnolence and disorientation with physostigmine. Anaesthesiology 44: 249, 1976.

4. Popescu, D.T.: Clinical experience with Etomidate. In: Anaesthesia and Pharmacology. Boerhaave series No. 12. Leiden. Leiden University Press, p. 151 (1976).

5. Lonneux, Y., Dinc, P., Royer, Ph., Moerman, E., Keersmakers, R., Driesens, F.: Alfentanyl, a new very short-acting analgesic during anaesthesia. Lecture presented at the 7th World Congress Hamburg. 16 September 1980.

ETOMIDATE AND OTHER NEW INDUCTION AGENTS

A. DOENICKE, Th. DUKA

General anaesthesia in adults involves induction with intravenous agents. In addition, intravenous agents are often
given in small repeated doses to maintain sleep and these
represent one of the components of what is called "balanced"
anaesthesia. With this technique the anaesthetic induction
agent is usually combined with nitrous oxide, potent analgesics and/or muscle relaxants. Ideally an agent which
could serve for induction and maintenance should fulfil the
following criteria: 1. cause rapid loss of consciousness,
2. be rapidly metabolised and excreted, 3. produce rapid and
smooth emergence, 4. be readily accepted by the patient,
5. be devoid of cardiovascular and/or respiratory adverse
effects, 6. cause a minimum of pain or irritation at the
site of injection, and 7. show compatibility with other intravenous agents. In this report we will present and discuss experimental data concerning certain of the advantages and disadvantages of some currently used and newly developed anaesthetic agents.

Etomidate, first investigated in animal studies by Paul
Janssen in 1971, was shown to be a potent, short acting hypnotic agent (20). Etomidate is an imidazole carboxylate which
is rapidly metabolised in the liver, and consequently has a
short duration of action. In rats its potency was shown to
be approximately 6 times greater than propanidid, its safety
margin is 26, whereas methohexitone and thiopentone show safety margins of 9 and 4 respectively (20). After extensive and
successful animal experiments, the drug was first administered
to patients in our department in 1972. During these trials
intra-arterial blood pressure, heart rate and respiration were

50

continously monitored. The appearance of myocloni, increase
of heart rate, involuntary defensive movements and other signs
of insufficient anaesthesia convinced us not to continue using
etomidate alone in subsequent clinical trials. Rather, we
undertook a series of studies utilizing volunteers to elucidate
the effect of etomidate on several parameters. Since it is established that many anaesthetic agents produce a release of
histamine, we were particularly interested in examining the
effect of etomidate on this variable. In experiments performed
with volunteers, etomidate was compared with three other hypnotics (methohexitone, althesin, propanidid) with respect to
their effects on plasma histamine levels; these studies showed
that only etomidate did not elicit a release of histamine
(Fig. 1) (13).

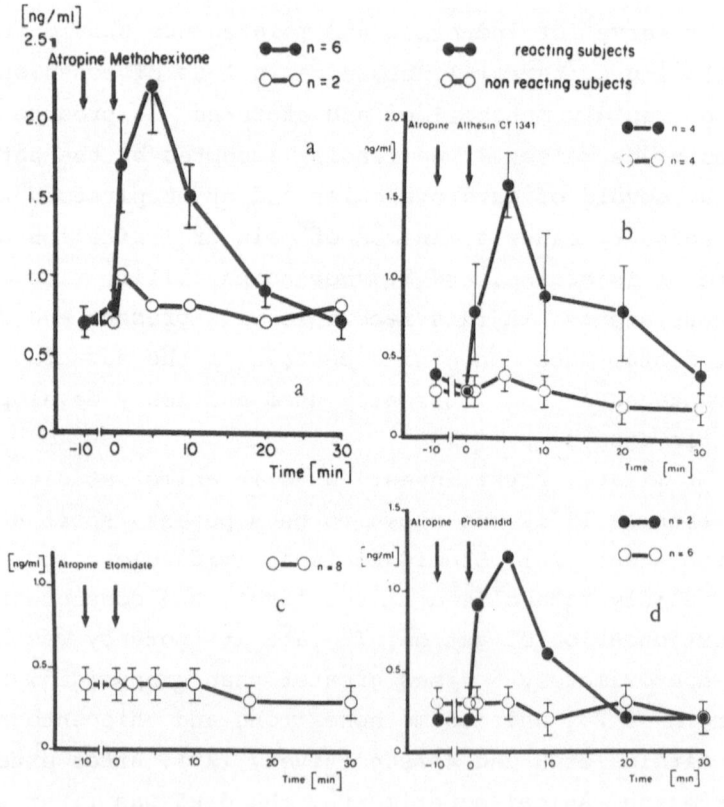

Fig. 1: Plasma histamine concentrations in volunteers after
i.v. administration of methohexitone (a), althesin (b),
etomidate (c), propanidid (d).

The effects of etomidate and propanidid on blood pressure were examined and compared in another investigation. It was observed that etomidate had no effect on circulation, whereas propanidid produced a decrease in the systolic blood pressure of approx. 25% (Fig. 2), (8).

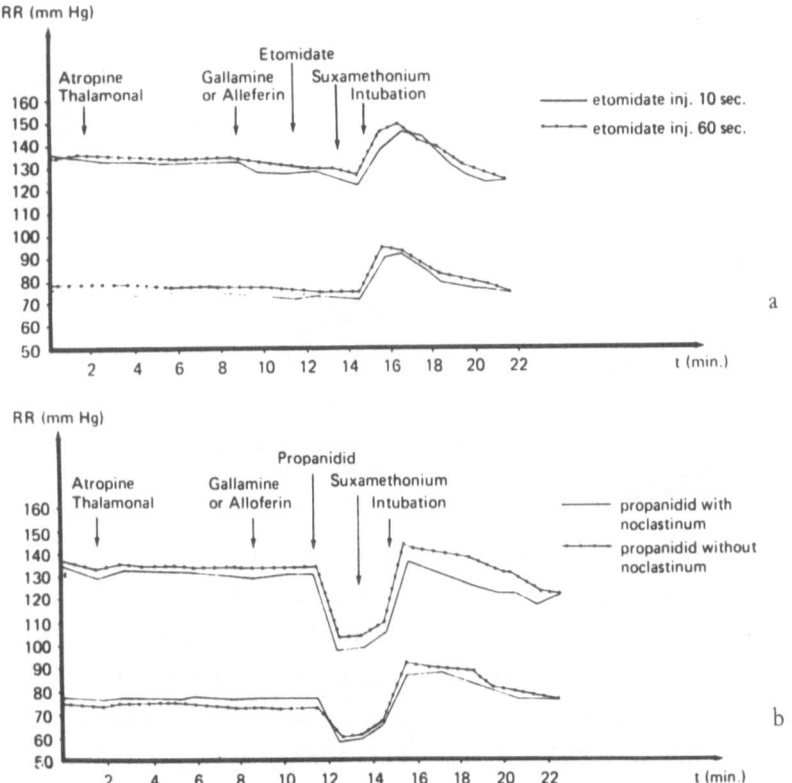

Fig. 2: Blood pressure during induction phase (a) with etomidate 0.15 mg/kg (inj.speed 10 s, n = 43, inj.speed 60 s = 37) and (b) with propanidid 0.5 mg/kg (with neclastinum, n = 31; without neclastinum, n = 73)

Another experimental procedure was carried out to compare the effects of etomidate, methohexital and propanidid on respiratory changes. In these experiments each subject received each of the drugs on different days separated by intervals of two weeks. With methohexital, the blood gas analyses showed a significant increase in the PCO_2 (partial pressure CO_2), and a significant drop in the PO_2 (partial pressure O_2) (Fig. 3a + b) (14).

52

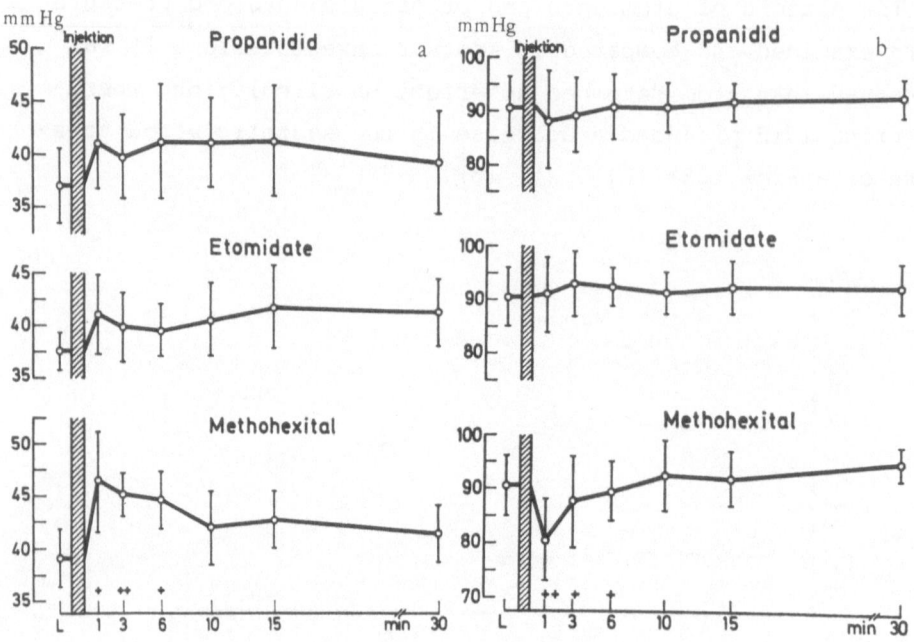

Fig. 3: a) CO_2 partial pressure (mmHg) n = 12
b) O_2 partial pressure (mmHg) N = 12
with different induction agents

At the given dosages, no differences in the blood gases could
be detected with either propanidid or etomidate (Fig. 3a + b).
However, with higher doses of etomidate e.g. 0.3 mg/kg a decrease in PO_2 was observed, as has been also reported by Hempel-
man et al. (17). Blood sugar levels, serum cholinesterase activity and fat metabolism did not significantly change after any
of the three hypnotics (9).

We further investigated the hypnotic effect of etomidate
utilising the electroencephalogram (eeg). These experiments were
performed in healthy volunteers. The eeg was taken from two
longitudinal rows of electrodes situated paramedially and recorded in 8 channels. Simultaneously with the monitoring of the
eeg, electrocardiogram, oculogram, spirogram, pneumotachogram,
body temperature and peripheral circulation were recorded and
CO_2, O_2 concentrations, in end tidal volumes were continously
measured. The eeg curves were evaluated visually and classified
according to the eeg stages in each successive 40 sec period (22).
These values were plotted in a compressed time scale to generate

"hypnograms". "Hypnograms" represent the depth of sleep over a period of testing. After etomidate injection, the "hypnogram" showed a rapid transition from the conscious to the deep anaesthetic stages, with max. effect obtained by 2 min after the injection (Fig. 4).

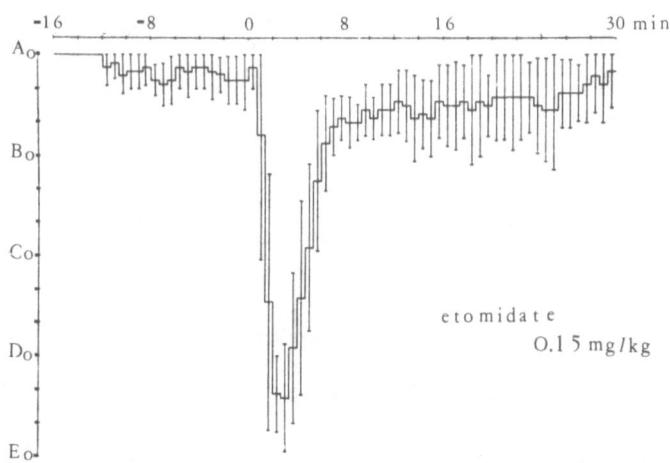

Fig. 4: "Hypnogram" after etomidate 0.15 mg/kg injected i.v. in 60 s (drug was injected at 0 time) n = 8

Within 3 to 4 minutes from the time of injection, deep anaesthesia stages were followed by the postanaesthetic oscillation of vigilance (Fig. 4, Fig. 5).

The most striking side effect with etomidate was myoclonic movement. This undesirable side effect happened less frequently after strong premedication. It is noteworthy that paroxysmal potentials were never detected in the eeg during these events. Furthermore, several patients suffering from epilepsy were given etomidate while their eeg was monitored and there were no complications (23). Preliminary data from our laboratory suggest that diazepam (0.07 mg/kg) when administered before etomidate (0.15 mg/kg) not only significantly reduced the incidence of myoclonic movement but also considerably prolonged the duration of sleep.

54

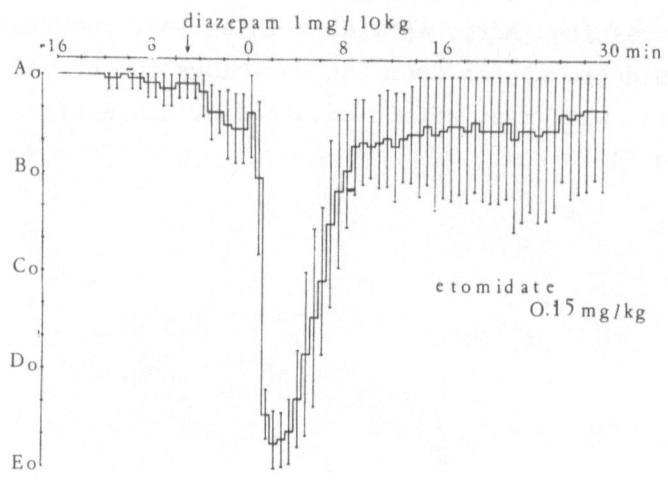

Fig. 5:
"Hypnogram" after etomidate 0.15 mg/kg injected i.v. in 60 s
with diazepam 1 mg/10 kg as premedication drug
(etomidate was injected at 0 time) n = 9

Since diazepam has been shown to have certain undesirable side
effects, such as thrombophlebitis and a long lasting hypnotic
effect as well as hangover (probably because of its metabolism
to active metabolites), two new benzodiazepine derivatives,
flunitrazepam (Ro-54000) and lormetazepam (SHF 12) were tested
(10). In these studies, flunitrazepam showed a longer duration
of sleep and also a decrease of PO_2 as compared to lormetazepam
(Fig. 6a + b). Consequently we continued these investigations
by comparing only diazepam and etomidate with lormetazepam and
etomidate (12). From the eeg it was observed that the hypnotic
effect of etomidate decreased more rapidly when lormetazepam was
given as premedication (Fig. 7a + b). No side effects were observed with lormetazepam, whereas six out of ten subjects got
thrombophlebitis after diazepam. No apnoea or respiratory depression occurred after lormetazepam combined with etomidate,
whereas changes of the PO_2 were found after diazepam with
etomidate.

Another side effect of the etomidate was pain at the site
of injection. One way to avoid this is to inject an opiate
analgesic e.g. fentanyl, shortly before administering etomidate.

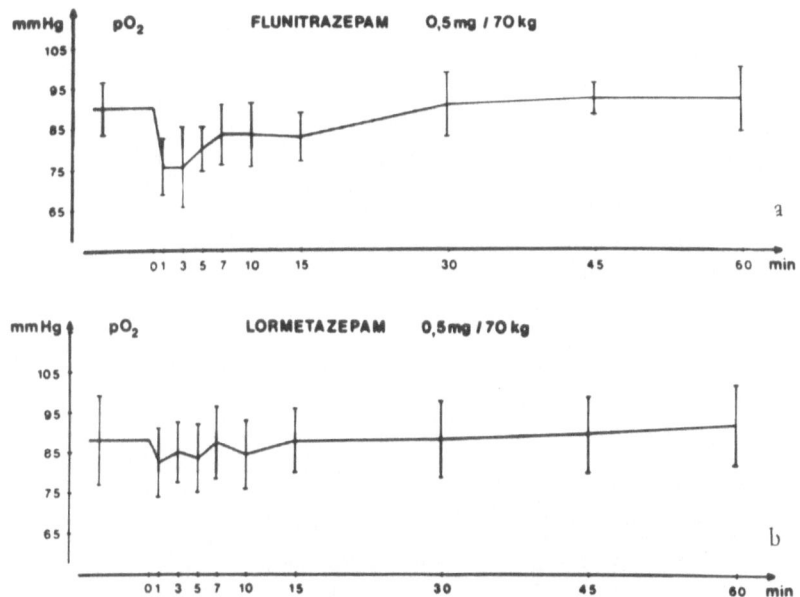

Fig. 6: O$_2$ partial pressure
a) after flunitrazepam injection 0.5 mg/70 kg, n = 12
b) after lormetazepam injection 0.5 mg/70 kg, n = 12

This additionally offers an analgesic for the operation since etomidate does not retain any analgesic action. The safe use of etomidate in the clinic clearly required further investigations. During the course of long operations, for instance, the substance has to be repeatedly administered in order to maintain anaesthesia. Thus a detailed knowledge of drug plasma levels, after various mode of administration, is necessary (4). However, a correlation of plasma levels with the desirable effect would be more instructive for this purpose. Using the method described by Wynants et al. (28), we measured plasma levels of etomidate and correlated these with its hypnotic effect by evaluating the eeg. The study was performed on two groups of volunteers. In the first group, 0.3 mg/kg etomidate was administered as a bolus injection, whereas in the second group this injection was followed at 4 and 8 min by injections of 0.15 mg/kg (Fig.8a + b). As premedication, fentanyl (0.1 mg) and diazepam (0.05 mg/kg) were administered at 5 and 10 minutes prior to etomidate injec-

56

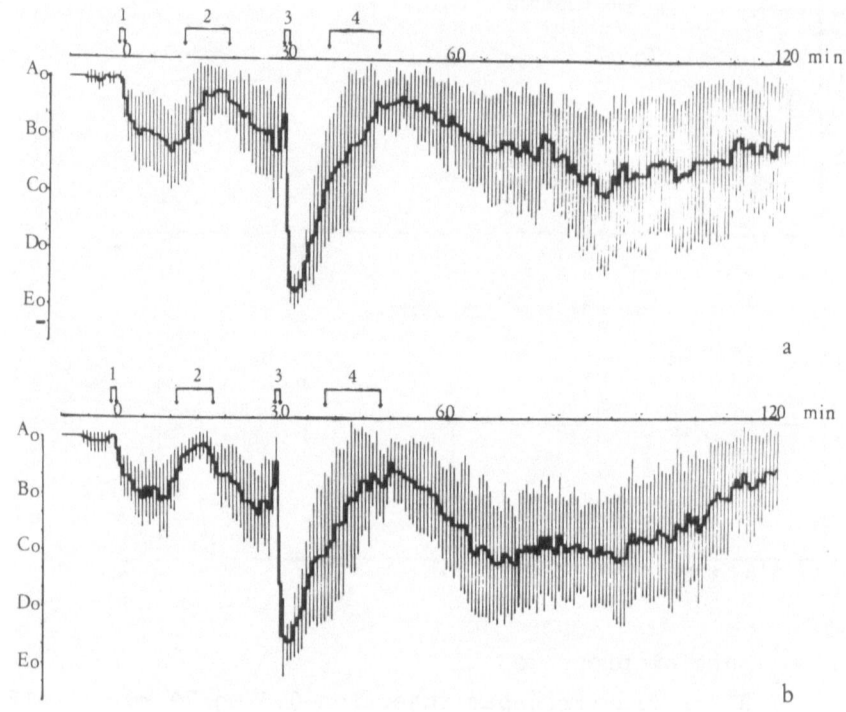

a

b

Fig. 7: "Hypnogram" after etomidate 0.15 mg/kg

    a) when diazepam 10 mg/70 kg, n = 10
    b) when lormetazepam 1 mg/70 kg, n = 10

    is given as premedication drug.

    Numbers given on the figure indicate
    1: diazepam or lormetazepam injection
    2: time during which patient is asked whether he was
       subjected to histamine release symptoms
    3: etomidate injection
    4: time during which patient is asked whether he was
       subjected to histamine release symptoms

    It can be seen that deeper sleep stages are reached
    when lormetazepam is given as a premedication drug;
    the duration of the effect is shorter.

tion respectively (9). In both groups there was a good correlation between the plasma levels of the drug and the hypnotic
effect (Fig. 8, Fig. 9).

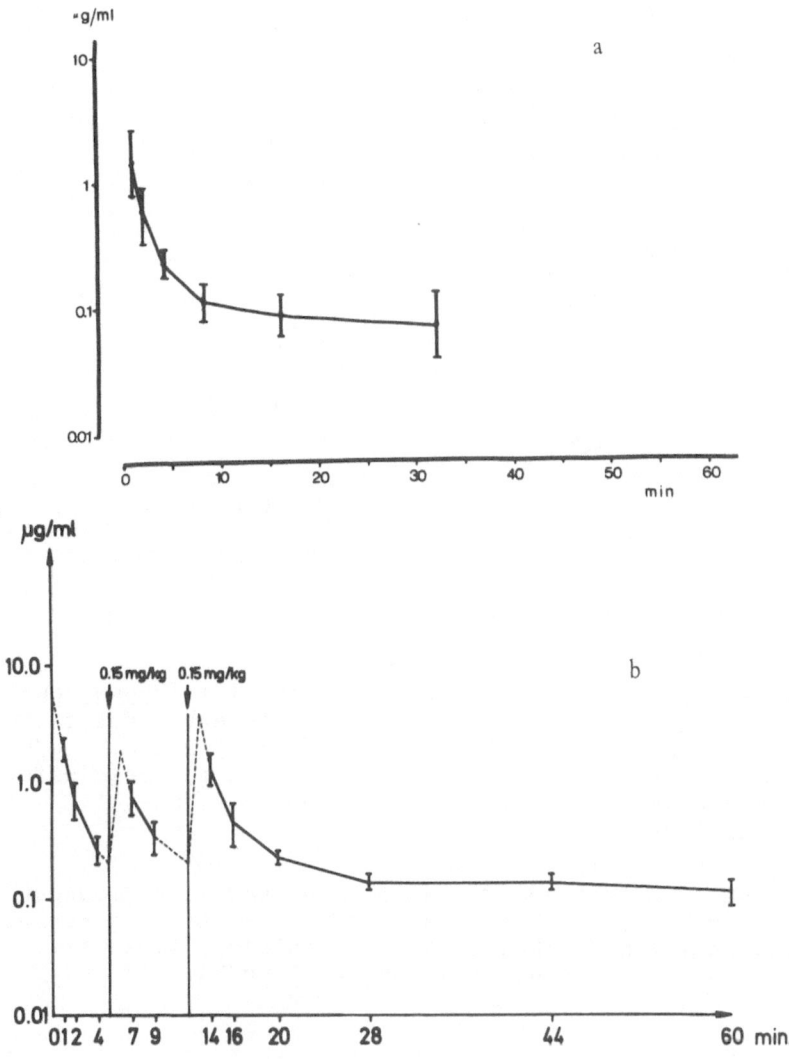

Fig. 8: Etomidate plasma concentrations after an i.v. injection of 0.3 mg/kg (n = 6) (a), and an i.v. injection of 0.3 mg/kg followed by two injections of
0.15 mg/kg at 5 and 10 min (b) (n = 6).

58

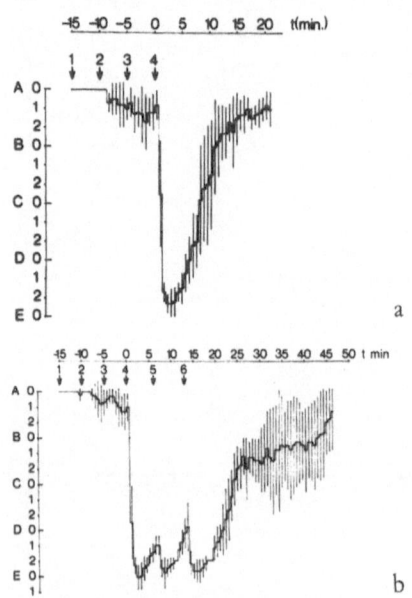

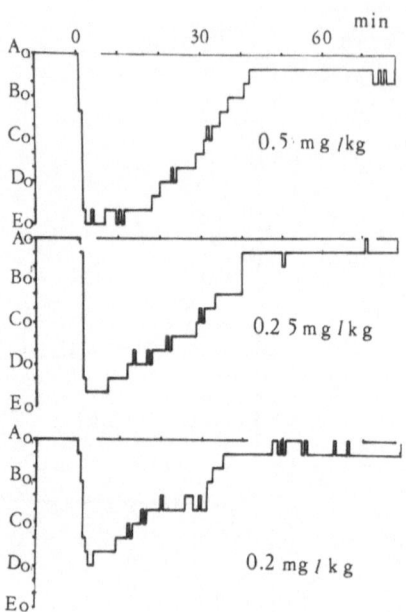

Fig. 9: "Hypnogram" after etomidate bolus injection 0.3
mg/kg (a) (n = 6) and after 3
repetitive injections of etomidate and two injections of
0,15 mg/kg at 5 and 10 min (b)
(n = 6).

Fig. 10: "Hypnograms" after
different doses of minaxolon
(0.5, 0.25, 0.2 mg/kg).
A dose response effect can
be seen (n = 3).

Atropine, diazepam and fentanyl were used as premedication
drugs. Numbers, given in the figure indicate 1: atropine 0.5 mg,
2: diazepam 1 mg/10 kg, 3: 0.1 mg fentanyl, 4: etomidate
0.3 mg/kg and 5 and 6: etomidate 0.15 mg/kg.

Steroid anaesthetics represent another group of drugs for
induction and maintenance of anaesthesia. Althesin, the main
representative of this class of drugs has to be formulated in
a solution containing cremophor EL which is known to cause anaphylactoid reactions (4). Thus, minaxolon, a new steroid anaesthetic which is water soluble, appeared to be promising. Experiments in laboratory animals have shown minaxolon to be a
potent (three times more than althesin and eight times more than
thiopental), rapidly acting anaesthetic with a higher safety
margin than althesin (3). From preliminary clinical experiments

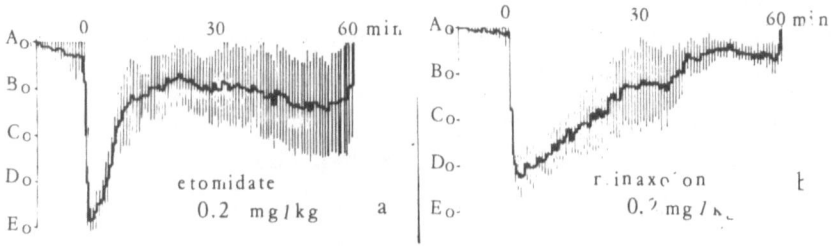

Fig. 11: "Hypnograms" after etomidate 0.2 mg/kg (n = 5) (a) and
after minaxolon 0.2 mg/kg (n= 5) (b).
With etomidate deeper sleep stages are reached and
shorter duration of the hypnotic effect is obtained.

minaxolon was demonstrated to be a very useful agent for induction and maintenance of anaesthesia (1).

Before using minaxolon in the clinic, we were interested in
estimating the optimal dose of the drug. Utilising volunteers,
we thus studied the eeg changes produced by the drug. In a preliminary investigation, several doses of minaxolon (0.20, 0.25,
0.5 mg/kg) were given and the changes in the depth of sleep
were studied from the "hypnograms" (Fig. 10).
When minaxolon was injected, some excitatory effects (hyper-
tonous, cough and hiccough,) were observed. The results of a
comparison study between etomidate and minaxolon are seen in
Fig. 11. The hypnotic effect of minaxolon showed a longer duration than etomidate, while the peak effects appear to be the
same for both substances. In the respiratory as well as in the
cardiovascular system, neither substance showed any significant
effect. However, recent toxicological experiments have shown
that it is carcinogenic in a certain species of mice. The company has subsequently withdrawn the drug from clinical research.

Benzodiazepines, with their benign cardiorespiratory effects
and reasonably rapid onset of action have provided an alternative to barbiturates as anaesthetic induction agents. Diazepam in particular has been used to induce anaesthesia where
thiopental is contraindicated, e.g. in the presence of por-

phyria (19), shock or limited cardiac reserve (7). However, the long duration of action (18) and the non aequous preparation (24), have limited its use. Primarily due to the low solubility of diazepam, an intense search has been made for a water soluble benzodiazepine. Midazolam is such a compound.

Midazolam in animal studies has shown benzodiazepine like pharmacological effects. From clinical studies (6) in which midazolam was used as either premedication drug or to produce anaesthesia, this drug was shown to be an excellent premedication drug, and an effective alternative of thiopental or etomidate for the induction of anaesthesia. Similar results were obtained in other clinical studies (5). When compared with diazepam for the induction of anaesthesia, midazolam was one and a half times more potent and, in addition, was more rapid in action (25). Moreover, pharmacological work has indicated that midazolam has minimal cardiovascular effects (26).

We examined the effects of midazolam on volunteers using eeg as a methodological tool to assess the hypnotic effect and the pharmacodynamics of the drug. The optimal dose was found by performing an analysis of the eeg when midazolam was injected i.v. in several doses (0.025, 0.05, 0.075, 0.1, 0.125, 0.15 mg/kg) (16). Even with the smallest dose used, a depth of sleep up to the B_2 stage was obtained (Fig. 12). With increasing dosages, an increase of depth of sleep (C_o stage) and of the duration of sleep stages (50 min) was observed (Fig. 12). In addition the effect of midazolam at a fixed dosage (0.10 mg/kg) was examined by injecting the substance over different periods of time (15 or 60 s) (Fig. 13) (11). The short time injection shows a more rapid onset as well as a shorter duration of the hypnotic effect. As can be seen in Fig. 13, 20 min after the short time injection stages of postanaesthetic vigilance have already been reached whereas with the 60 s injection, middle or even deep sleep stages were still taking place. Cardiovascular effects with midazolam were minimal.

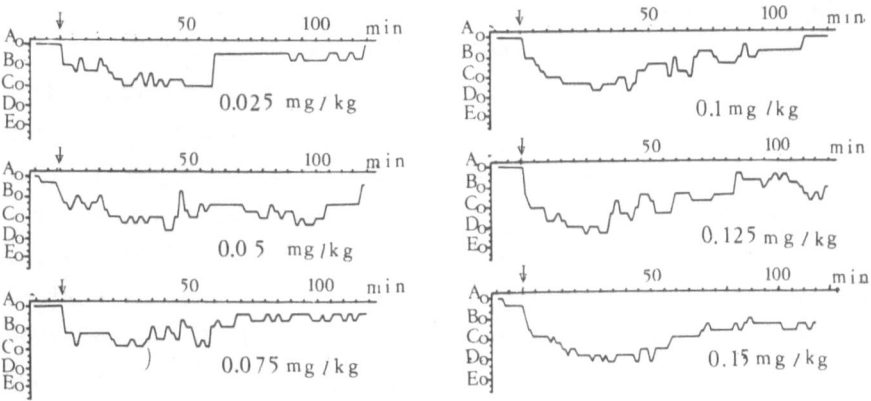

Fig. 12: "Hypnograms" after different doses of midazolam,
n = 3. The arrows indicate the time of injection.

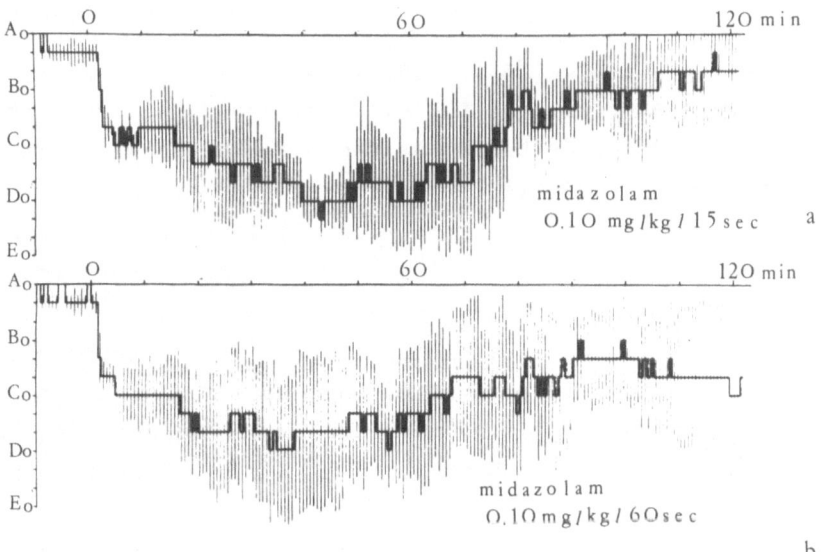

Fig. 13: "Hypnograms" after midazolam 0.10 mg/kg injected in
15 s (a) (n = 6) and in 60 s (b) (n = 6).
The duration of the effect in 60 min injection is
clearly longer.

Diprivan is another new anaesthetic which we have recently
investigated. Structurally, it is unrelated to other induction
substances. Its solubility in water is low and it is therefore

necessary to make solutions of this drug in cremophor. Use
of this drug in animal studies (15) and in preliminary clinical trials (21, 27) has given promising results, but a detailed
dose response curve of the drug has not as yet been performed.
By using in our laboratory different doses of diprivan (1.5,
1.75, 2.0 mg/kg) on volunteers, reliable sleep stages were
reached following doses of 1.5 mg/kg and above (Fig. 14), with
the maximum effect lasting about 3 to 4 min (which is similar
to the effect of etomidate). With 2.0 mg/kg, the highest dose
we tested, the maximal sleep depth reached was E_o, with the
maximum effect lasting 3 to 4 min (Fig. 14). Apart from occasional, slight injection pain, which was not associated with redde-
ning or venous irritation, no side effects were observed. Cardiovascular parameters remained constant apart from slight
decreases in blood pressure and heart rate.

In conclusion, etomidate after 9 years of investigation, is
perhaps the most useful of the available anaesthetic agents
for a "balanced" anaesthesia. As shown in the initial clinical
trials etomidate exhibits the following side effects:
1. pain at the site of the injection, 2. lack of analgesia, and
3. myoclonia. Nevertheless, it possesses certain very important
advantages: 1. short duration of action, 2. no signs of hangover
either after bolus or after infusion, and 3. no anaphylactoid
reaction. Additionally etomidate, when compared with other intravenous anaesthetics (e.g. althesin, ketamine, methohexital,
propanidid, thiopental and droperidol) has been shown to produce only very small effects on haemodynamics and no significant changes on myocardial blood flow and myocardial oxygen
consumption (2, 17). Even on combination with an analgesic, e.g.
fentanyl, piritramid does not show any cardiovascular changes,
which is especially important in patients with coronary artery
disease. It is worthwhile to note that myoclonia are completely
antagonised when benzodiazepines (especially lormetazepam) are
given as premedication drugs.

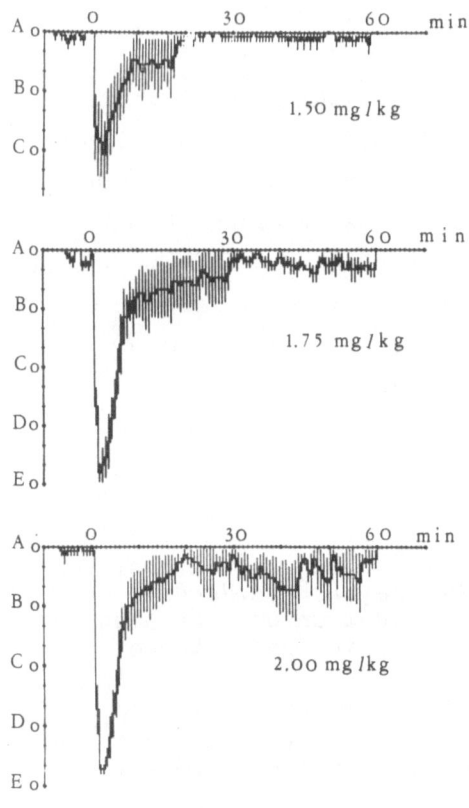

Fig. 14:
"Hypnogram" after
different doses of
diprivan (1.5, 1.75,
2.0 mg/kg) (each n = 5)

Concerning minaxolon, initial experimental investigations
have demonstrated it to be a very interesting substance for
anaesthesia. It exerts a longer hypnotic effect than etomidate
but does not show any cardiovascular changes. In addition no
irritation was observed in the site of the injection. However,
since the toxicological effects of the substance have not yet
been clarified, the substance has been withdrawn from clinical
research.

Midazolam, a new benzodiazepine derivative, takes a special
place among benzodiazepines because of its characteristic of
water solubility. It shows a rapid onset of the hypnotic effect
and a short functional half life. Deep sleep stages are reached
within a few minutes such that the mode of hypnotic effect
resembles that of the classic anaesthetic agent thiopental.

Cardiovascular side effects are minimal.

Diprivan, which is still under clinical investigation, shows a rapid onset of the hypnotic effect and a short half life. When administered via infusion in combination with N_2O diprivan appears to be ideal for the maintenance of anaesthesia, however, the primary disadvantage remains the solution cremophor EL in which the substance must be dissolved. In our experiments when high doses were used, flush, a sign of histamine release, was often observed.

REFERENCES

1. Aveling,W., J.W.Sear, W.Fitch, H.Chang, A.Waters, Gm.Cooper, P.Simpson, T.M.Savege, L.Prys,Roberts, D.Campbell: Early clinical evaluation of minaxolon. A new intravenous steroid anaesthetic agent. Lancet (in press) (1980)

2. Brückner,J.B., J.W.Gethmann, D.Patschke, J.Tarnow, A.Weymar: Untersuchungen zur Wirkung von Etomidate auf den Kreislauf des Menschen. Anaesthesist 23,322 (1974)

3. Child,K.J., J.P.Currie, Dodds,D.B., D.R.Pearse, D.J.Twissell: The pharmacological properties in animals of CT 1341. A new steroid anaesthetic agent. Br.J. Anaesthesia 43, 2 (1971

4. Choneim,M.M. and K.Kortille: Pharmacokinetics of intravenous anaesthetics implications for clinical use. Clin.Pharmacokin. 2,344 (1977)

5. Colin R.Brown, F.H.Sarnquist, C.A.Canup, T.Pedley: Clinical electroencephalographic and pharmacokinetic studies of a water soluble benzodiazepine: Midazolam maleate. Anaesthesiology 50, 467 (1979)

6. Conner,J.T., R.L.Katz, R.R.Pagano, W.C.Graham: Ro 21-3981 for intravenous surgical premedication and induction of anaesthesia. Anaesth.Analg. 57, 1 (1978)

7. Dalen,J.E., G.L.Evans, J.S.Banas: The haemodynamic and respiratory effects of diazepam. Anaesthesiology 30, 259 (1969)

8. Doenicke,A.: Etomidate, a new intravenous hypnotic. Acta anaesth.belg. 25,307 (1974)

9. Doenicke,A.: Klinische Pharmakologie in: Lehrbuch der Anaesthesiologie. Reanimation und intensive Therapie. Hrsg. H.Benzer, R.Frey, W.Higin, O.Mayhofer. Springer Verlag Berlin (1977)

10. Doenicke,A., J.Kugler, M.Kropp, M.Laub, G.Kalbfleisch: Der hypnotische Effekt des neuen Benzodiazepinderivats Lormetazepam nach intravenöser Injektion. Anaesthesist, **28**, 578 (1979)

11. Doenicke,A., J.Kugler, H.Suttmann, B.Grote, W.Donner: Midazolam: Abhängigkeit der Schlaftiefe von Injektionszeit und Dosis. Anaesthesist, **29**, 636 (1980)

12. Doenicke,A., W.Lorenz, J.Dittmann, P.Hug, E.Hinterlang: Histaminfreisetzung nach Diazepam/Lormetazepam in Kombination mit Etomidate. (Workshop Einbeck 1978), in: Lormetazepam. Hrsg. A.Doenicke, H.Ott. Anaesthesiologie u.Intensivmed. 133, Springer, Bln.-Heidelbg.-New York

13. Doenicke,A., Lorenz,W.,R.Beigl, H.Bezecny, G.Uhlig, L. Kalmar, B.Praetorius, G.Mann: Histamine release after intravenous application of short acting hypnotics. A comparison of Etomidate, Althesin (T 1341)and Propanidid Brit.J.Anaesth. **45**, 1097 (1973)

14. Doenicke,A., E.Wagner, K.H.Beetz: Blutgasanalysen (arteriell) nach drei kurzwirkenden i.v. Hypnotika (Propanidid, Etomidate, Methohexital). Anaesthesist 22,353(1973)

15. Glen,J.B.: Animal studies of the anaesthetic activity of ICI 35868, Br.J.Anaesth. **52**, 743 (1980)

16. Grote,B., A.Doenicke, J.Kugler, H.Suttmann, M.Laub: Midazolam: Dosisfindung mit Hilfe des Encephalogramms. Anaesthesist **29**, 635 (1980)

17. Hempelmann,W., Hempelmann,G., Piepenbrock,S.: A comparative study of blood gases and haemodynamics using the new hypnotic etomidate,CT 1341, methohexitone, propanidid and thiopentone; in: Etomidate , ed. by A.Doenicke. Springer-Verlag, Berlin-Heidelberg-New York (1977)

18. Hillstad,L., T.Hansen, H.Melsom: Diazepam metabolism in normal man. Clin.Pharm.Ther. **16**, 479 (1974)

19. Jackson,S.H.: Genetic and metabolic disease hereditary hepatic porphyrias. Anaesthesia and uncommon diseases. Pathophysiologic and clinical correlations, ed.by Katz, J. and L.B.Kadis. Philadelphia W.B. Saunders 10 (1973)

20. Janssen,P.A.J., Niemegeers,C.J.E., Schellekens,K.H.L., Lenaerts,F.M.: Etomidate, R (+)Ethyl-1-(alpha-methyl-benzyl) imidazole-5-carboxylate (R 16 659), a potent, short acting relatively atoxic intravenous hypnotic agent in rats. Arzneimittel-Forsch. **21**, 1234 (1971)

21. Kay,B. and G.Rolly: ICI 35868, a new intravenous induction agent. Acta Anaesth.Belg. **28**, 303 (1977)

22. Kugler,J.: Electroencephalographie in Klinik und Praxis. Georg Thieme Verlag, Stuttgart, 1966.

23. Kugler,J., A.Doenicke, M.Laub: The EEG after Etomidate, in: Etomidate. Ed.by A.Doenicke. Anaesthesiologie **106**, 31 (1977). Springer-Verlag, Berlin-Heidelberg-New York

24. Langdom,D.E., J.R.Harlan, R.L.Bailey: Thrombophlebitis
    with diazepam used intravenously. JAMA 223, 184 (1973)

25. Reves,J.G., G.Corssen , C.Holcob: Comparison of two
    benzodiazepines for anaesthesia induction: Midazolam
    and Diazepam. Canad.Anaesth.Soc.J. 25, 211 (1978)

26. Reves,J.G., M.Mardie: Cardiovascular effects of Ro 213
    981, Fed.proc. 37 (3) Abstr. 1548 (1978)

27. Rogers,K.M., K.M.S.Dewar, T.D.McCubbin, A.A.Spence:
    Preliminary experience with ICI 35868 as an I.V. induc-
    tion agent. Comparison with althesin. Br.J.Anaesth. 52,
    807 (1980)

28. Wynants,J., R.Woestenborghs, J.Heykants: A gas chromato-
    graphic assay method for etomidate in human plasma.
    Biological research reports. Janssen Pharmaceutica
    Dex. 1974

OPIOID RECEPTORS AND ANALGESIA

A. Witter

1. INTRODUCTION

Opioids or opioid agonists can be designated generically as
substances that bind specifically to any of the opioid receptors and produce some agonistic action. The term opioid has more or less displaced the
word opiate, that in a more strict sense refers to drugs derived from
opium, the juice of the poppy Papaver somniferum, like morphine.

Drugs like morphine interact with receptors to produce biochemical
alterations of cell function and ultimately elicit a pharmacological response. However, since exogenous drugs are plant products or man-made synthetic
substances, it is obvious that evolution has not developed specific receptors
for them. These receptors, with which most drugs interact, actually represent
receptors for endogenous substances. These endogenous substances play a
physiological role in the normal functioning of an organism. Exogenous drugs
mimic the actions of endogenous substances and can thus be applied during
pathological conditions or to create extreme functioning of an organism, as
for example to suppress severe pain.

About ten years ago the existence of stereospecific opioid binding sites
was demonstrated, enhancing the likelihood of the presence of endogenous
opioid substances. These sites were located in the brain and since many,
but not all, opioid activities are of central origin it seemed a logical
approach to use the brain as the starting material in the search for endogenous
opioids. A prerequisite for the isolation of endogenous compounds is the
availability of a suitable assay system, guiding the purification of the
assumed endogenous opioid. Assay systems that played a dominant role in the
detection and measurement of endogenous opioids were a bio-assay (the guinea
pig ileum preparation) and a radiochemical assay: the radioligand assay,
also called radioreceptor assay.

2. THE RADIORECEPTOR ASSAY

In an in vitro ligand binding assay, a crude tissue preparation from the target tissue - in this case the brain - is used, because it can be expected to contain the hypothetical receptor together with numerous other tissue and cell constituents. As ligands, radioactive labeled agonists, like ^{3}H-dihydromorphine, or antagonists, like ^{3}H-naloxone are used. After incubation to equilibrium of the radioactively labeled ligand with the crude tissue preparation, the bound and free ligand are separated and the bound ligand is counted for radioactivity. This represents the total bound ligand, that is ligand bound both to the receptor and to non-receptor components present in the crude tissue preparation. To differentiate between receptor and non-receptor binding, the incubation is repeated in the presence of a 100-1000 fold excess of non-labeled ligand. This will displace virtually all radio-actively labeled ligand from those binding sites that originally were practically completely occupied. If, as is usual, the concentration of the labeled ligand is in the order of 10^{-9}M, almost complete occupation will occur only with sites characterized by low capacity (in the order of 10^{-10}M) and high affinity (K_{diss} in the order of 10^{-10}M) for the labeled ligand. These properties are usually fulfilled by receptor binding sites. In contrast, only a small fraction of the high capacity, low affinity sites will be occupied by the labeled ligand, and the addition of an excess of non-labeled ligand will not result in displacement but in the occupation of hitherto unoccupied sites. Therefore, in the presence of an excess of non-labeled ligand, the amount bound represents the non-displacable binding sites. The difference between the amount bound in the absence and presence of an excess of non-labeled ligand thus represents displacable binding. Comparison of various non-labeled ligands should yield a positive correlation between their in vivo potencies to elicit a pharmacological response (allowing for differences in availability for receptor interactions) and their in vitro potencies to displace the labeled ligand: structural and steric specificity. The location of the binding sites should be discrete and correlate with target tissue specificity. If these criteria, together with the earlier defined saturability (limited number of sites) and high affinity (consistent with physiological/pharmacological agonist concentration), are fulfilled, the displacable binding can be re-evaluated as specific binding. Simultaneous correlations of in vitro binding directly with a biochemical event associated with the pharmacological response and parallel changes of binding-

and biological properties after (bio)chemical manipulations of the binding sites finally allow characterization of the binding as true <u>receptor binding</u>. Besides the differentiation between specific (displacable) and non-specific (non-displacable) binding, a further distinction has to be made for a number of ligands, especially the larger polypeptides. This refers to specific binding and the differentiation is between specific receptor binding and specific non-receptor binding. The latter is often characterized by high affinity, low capacity, reversibility and even structural specificity, and represents specific binding to tube walls, filters and such in the absence of receptor tissue. The presence of specific non-receptor binding has to be verified and, if present, the specific non-receptor sites have to be occupied by inert compounds, like serum albumine, before specific receptor assays can be carried through.

Despite these limitations, the radioligand assay has been a helpful tool in the isolation of endogenous opioids. Radioactively labeled opioid agonists or antagonists are incubated with brain tissue preparations, containing the opioid "receptor", in the absence or presence of purified brain extracts, containing the endogenous opioids. Endogenous opioids in the purified brain fractions manifest themselves by displacing the specific "receptor"-bound, radioactively labeled exogenous opioid agonist or antagonist. From 1975 onward a number of endogenous opioids have been isolated from brain and pituitary extracts and their structures determined.

3. ENDOGENOUS OPIOIDS (ENDORPHINS)
3.1. The enkephalins

The first to be discovered were the enkephalins, two pentapeptides Met-enkephalin and Leu-enkephalin, that differ only in one amino acid (the C-terminal). Met-enkephalin is identical to the amino acid sequence 61-65 of the pituitary hormone β-LPH (β-lipotropin). Available evidence suggests that β-LPH is probably not the (only) immediate precursor for enkephalin. Leu-enkephalin is one of the endogenous opioid peptides whose sequence is not part of β-LPH, because of the presence of the Leu^{65} residue and this seems to rule out β-LPH as a precursor molecule. Recently, the isolation of a pentadecapeptide α-neo-endorphin (1) and a tridecapeptide dynorphin 1-13 (2,3) has been described. These polypeptides have the sequence of Leu-enkephalin at their N-termini and could function as potential precursor molecules. The remaining structure of these larger peptides is completely

different from that following the 61-65 sequence in β-LPH, indicating a
different origin. Subsequently, dynorphin 1-8 (4) and Leu-enkephalin-Arg-OH
(5) have been isolated from pituitary and hypothalamic extracts. A similar
situation appears to exist for Met-enkephalin. From the adrenal medulla,
where the presence of various larger putative pro-enkephalins as well as
relatively high amounts of enkephalin itself have been demonstrated (6,7),
a dodecapeptide BAM-12P has been isolated (8). This peptide shows some
structural resemblence to dynorphin and α-neo-endorphin. It appears that
BAM-12P is a C-terminal shortened peptide of a family of endogenous "big"
Met-enkephalins: BAM-20P and BAM-22P (9). The latter peptides are very
potent in the guinea pig ileum assay. From the adrenal, also the heptapeptide
Met-enkephalin-Arg-Phe-OH has been isolated (10), whereas Met(0)-enkephalin-
Arg-OH has been identified in porcine hypothalami (11). Finally, an analgesic
dipeptide H-Tyr-Arg-OH or kyotorphin has recently been isolated from bovine
brain (12). This peptide might act indirectly by releasing Met-enkephalin
and to some degree inhibiting enzymatic degradation of the released
enkephalin (13). The discovery of these peptides is not only interesting
from a genetic viewpoint, but also opens vista's for the development of
new analgesics. It seems possible that the adrenal opioid peptides play a
physiological role within the adrenal medulla itself rather than elsewhere,
because of their rapid degradation in plasma. This might take place through
action at an intracellular granular opioid receptor regulating the catecholamine content of the chromaffin granules (14). In subjects who died after
traffic accidents the post mortem opioid peptide levels in the adrenal
medullae were decreased about 10-fold as compared to persons who had died
from various internal diseases, possibly indicating massive premortal
adrenal medullary discharge (15).

3.2 The endorphins related to β-LPH

The second group of endogenous opioid peptides are the endorphins related
to β-LPH. The most potent in its opiate-like activity is β-endorphin, having
the sequence β-LPH 61-91. The hormone β-LPH is the immediate precursor of
β-endorphin. β-LPH has no opiate-like properties and is in turn derived
from a larger molecular weight precursor molecule, known as 31K, which also
contains the ACTH sequence. A number of smaller β-endorphin derived peptides
are also known to occur, like α-endorphin (β-LPH 61-76) and γ-endorphin
(β-LPH 61-77) (16).

4. IN VIVO FATE OF ENKEPHALINS AND ENDORPHINS

The in vivo pharmacological activity of drugs, for example the analgesic activity of opioids, is determined by various factors. These include the concentration of the opioid at the receptor, the concentration of the receptor, the interaction between opioid and receptor and the biochemical and ultimately pharmacological response resulting from this interaction. These aspects must be taken into account when new analgesics are to be developed.

The opioid concentration at the receptor sites is of course primarily dependent on the dosage and subsequently on the in vivo fate of the administered dose, i.c. its resorption, distribution and elimination (cf. following paper). For drugs acting in the CNS, the penetration through the blood-brain barrier and for drugs with a peptide structure the metabolic stability are of particular importance. It is generally agreed that passage of endogenous opioid peptides through the blood-brain barrier is severely restricted. Peripherally administered (iv) β-endorphin appears in the CSF, reaching a peak at about 1 hr after administration (17). The peak concentration in CSF is about 25% of the plasma level at that point in time; the peptide is cleared considerably faster from plasma than it is from CSF (18). The uptake in brain is restricted, with the possible exception of the hypothalamus (17,19). The much higher analgesic potency of β-endorphin after intracerebroventricular administration as compared to systemic administration (18) is in accordance with the observed restricted central uptake. Not only the hydrophilic character and high molecular weight of the opioid peptides appear responsible for this property, but also metabolic instability. The latter is particularly important in the case of the enkephalins. These peptides are metabolized extremely rapid in brain, where different enzyme systems appear to act (20): aminopeptidases hydrolyzing the H-Tyr-Gly- peptide bond, an enkephalinase A hydrolyzing the H-Tyr-Gly-Gly-Phe- linkage, an enkephalinase B hydrolyzing the H-Tyr-Gly-Gly- bond and carboxypeptidases removing the C-terminal amino acid methionine or leucine. Since most of the resulting metabolites are inactive, this catabolism is one of the main reasons for the low analgesic potency of enkephalins, even after intracerebroventricular administration. Various metabolically stable enkephalin derivatives have been synthesized which usually contain a D-Ala-2 residue together with some modification at position 5 (-D-Leu-5-OH, -Met-5-amide) (21). In contrast, β-endorphin is metabolically comparatively stable, probably because the secondary structure of this larger polypeptide protects its N-terminus - the enkephalin sequence - from the degrading enzymes. The properties mentioned above have a pronounced effect on the opioid concentration that becomes available for receptor interaction.

5. THE RECEPTORS

5.1. The opioid receptors

Another important factor concerns the nature and (local) concentration of the partner of the opioids, the opioid receptors. Although the opioids are used primarily as analgetics, they have many other effects as well. These limit their clinical use. Respiratory depression and the development of dependence, together with the induction of tolerance and the existence of an abstinence syndrome are among the most serious of these limiting side effects. Changes in mood and behavior, alterations of the endocrine system, decreased gastro-intestinal motility, miosis, nausea and emesis are other effects of the opioids. The mediation of these multiple effects can in part be explained by a lack of receptor selectivity, that is a certain receptor is located in different parts of the organism and coupled to effector systems that produce effects typical for the tissue involved, for example the CNS and the gastro-intestinal tract. There is also increasing evidence for a lack of receptor specificity, that is the action of a certain drug is not restricted to one distinct receptor, and different receptors are involved in the manifestation of multiple effects of a single drug. The existence of multiple opioid receptors is similar to the well-known distinction of α- and β-adrenergic receptors, muscarinic and nicotinic cholinergic receptors etc. Based on pharmacological evidence, the following opioid receptors were proposed: μ(mu)receptors for which morphine is the prototype agonist, κ(kappa)receptors acted upon by benzomorphans and δ(delta)receptors preferentially binding enkephalins (22,23,24,25, 26), although the existence of separate κ receptors has been questioned lately (27).

The structural requirements for the alkaloid opioid receptors focus on the spatial arrangement of the phenolic ring A, separated from a tertiary amine by two or three methylenes (28,29,30,31). Tyramine possesses these structural features, but is inactive as an opiate. Therefore additional binding sites, existing in the morphine molecule, are necessary. A model for the opiate receptor might contain a lipophilic site, interacting with

ring A, and an ionic site, interacting with the amine nitrogen. It is
generally accepted that the opiate receptor can exist in two conformations,
modulated by sodium ions. Under the prevailing sodium concentrations in the
brain, the opiate receptor probably exists predominantly in the antagonist
conformation. This conformation could be stabilized by interaction of a
specific antagonist receptor site with substituents in the opioid molecule
endowing it with antagonistic properties. At low sodium concentrations the
agonist conformation prevails. Obviously, binding of morphine also triggers
transformation to the agonist conformation, that could be stabilized by
the interaction of a specific receptor agonist site. The pharmacological
data used to derive such a model make it likely that this model describes
the μ receptor.

5.2. The enkephalin receptors

The discovery of endogenous opioid peptides further extended the concept
of multiple opioid receptors. The current hypothesis strongly favors the
existence of separate enkephalin or δ(delta)receptors and of preferential
endorphin or ϵ(epsilon)receptors. Some studies used opioid-sensitive
peripheral tissue preparations, the guinea pig ileum containing mainly
μ receptors and the mouse vas deferens containing predominantly δ receptors.
However, receptor heterogeneity has also been demonstrated in the CNS. The
enkephalins are distributed widely but unevenly throughout the brain, spinal
cord and peripheral autonomic nervous system. This distribution is closely
associated with the opiate receptor and CNS structures involved in the
regulation of sensory input such as pain perception. There is increasing
evidence that enkephalins act as neurotransmitters, in concord with their
rapid inactivation (cf. acetylcholine). Since brain function seems to be
encoded more in patterns of connectivity between nerve cells than in the
particular neurotransmitters employed by those nerve cells, the question
of the function of enkephalins cannot be translated into a simple answer.
Rather, enkephalins as neurotransmitters, or neuromodulators might participate
in many neuronal pathways, serving numerous physiological functions. The
opioid receptors identified in brain include μ-, δ- and recently β-endorphin
receptors.   The analgesic activity of opioids is usually connected with
μ receptors. These receptors are localized in areas, which are involved
preferentially in integrating sensory perception. They include layers 1
and 4 of the cerebral cortex and interneurons in the dorsal spinal cord,

synapsing on opioid receptors localized to nerve endings of sensory neurons. In the dorsal spinal cord enkephalins appear to inhibit the release of sensory "pain" neurotransmitters, as for example substance P, from these sensory nerve endings. On the other hand, the emotion-regulating limbic system is selectively enriched in δ receptors. It has been proposed that μ receptors interact preferentially with Met-enkephalin and δ receptors with Leu-enkephalin, because of parallel regional distributions in the brain (20).

At first sight, structural similarity between a complex molecule like morphine and the pentapeptide enkephalin might seem obscure. The basic requirements for opioid binding, however, are present in the N-terminal amino acid residue tyrosine. Indeed, des-Tyr-enkephalin and even desamino-Tyr[1]-enkephalin are biologically inactive. Initially, synthesis of enkephalin derivatives aimed at increasing metabolic stability, by for example replacing the Gly[2]-residue by a D-amino acid residue. The analgesic activity of D-Ala[2]- and D-Met[2]-enkephalins is similar to that of morphine after intracerebroventricular administration. A further increase in analgesic potency is obtained by also modifying the C-terminal residue; amidation of the C-terminal Leu- or Met-residue or substitution of Leu[5]-NH_2, or -Met[5]-NH_2 by Pro[5]-NH_2 enhance analgesic potency considerably. In most, but not in all cases, increased analgesic potency correlates with an increased affinity for μ receptors, both peripherally (guinea pig ileum) and centrally (displacement of specific ^{3}H-etorphine binding). Enkephalin analogs possessing high affinity for μ receptors relative to their affinity for δ receptors, for example D-Ala[2]-N-Me-Phe[4]-Met(O)-ol[5]-enkephalin, have been developed with potencies similar to that of morphine after oral or subcutaneous administration. The role of the Phe[4]-residue appears ambivalent. It might stabilize the agonist conformation for interaction with the μ receptor, but it also appears that the Phe[4]-residue is essential for binding to δ receptors, since replacement of the phenyl ring by an aliphatic hydrophobic moiety results in a complete loss of activity on the mouse vas deferens (δ receptors) whereas affinity for the μ receptors of the guinea pig ileum remains practically unchanged (32). Increased hydrophobicity, that is increased possibility of penetration through the blood-brain barrier, seems correlated mainly with an increased onset of analgesia. In this respect Leu[5]-enkephalins appear effective.

Besides these synthetic analogues, the naturally occurring C-terminally elongated enkephalins might hold promise for the future. Dynorphin, for example, is 12 times more potent in the guinea pig ileum preparation than in the mouse vas deferens, and its affinity for the peripheral μ receptor is considerably higher than that of enkephalin, normorphine or β-endorphin (2). It appears likely that dynorphin 1-13 interacts with specific opioid receptors in the mouse vas deferens, different from μ and δ receptors (33). Also D-Arg^6-dynorphin has affinity for this receptor, but not D-Ala^2-D-Arg^6-dynorphin. The CNS activities (analgesia, catatonia) of dynorphin are limited, probably because of its rapid in vivo degradation. However, D-Ala^2-dynorphin 1-11 is at least ten times more potent than dynorphin in analgesic activity after intracerebroventricular administration (34) and also D-Ala^2-D-Arg^6-dynorphin displays considerable antinociceptive activity (33). Similarly, Met-enkephalin-Arg-Phe-OH is about eight times more potent than Met-enkephalin (35).

5.3. The endorphin receptors

The distribution of the long-chain polypeptide β-endorphin in the CNS differs considerably from that of the enkephalins. β-Endorphin is present in a system that is centered around the hypothalamic-pituitary axis and extends in a defined pathway into the midline regions of the diencephalon and anterior pons. In contrast to the postulated neurotransmitter role of enkephalins, the action of β-endorphin tends to indicate a role in neuro-endocrine functioning. The relative metabolic stability and the slow dissociation from its binding site, findings that are congruent with the high potency and prolonged duration of action of β-endorphin, support such a function. The biological effects of β-endorphin reported until now are numerous, although often in need of unequivocal confirmation. These effects include analgesia, induction of tolerance, thermoregulation, regulation of respiration, limbic excitability, eating and central cardiovascular control, pituitary hormone-releasing activity and a role in learning and memory and in schizophrenia. It has been speculated that these effects might reflect an important role of β-endorphin in the corresponding physio-logical processes. In particular, a physiological role of β-endorphin in pain responses seems likely. The endorphin system is activated during pregnancy with a steep peak shortly before parturition, as has been inferred from rises in pain threshold (36,37). Electrical stimulation of the peri-ventricular and periaqueductal gray regions of the brain in humans suffering intractable pain results in a significant alleviation of the pain and a concomittant increase of β-endorphin levels in the CSF (38). There is also evidence that analgesia observed after electro-acupuncture is mediated by the release of β-endorphin into the CSF (39,40). Consequently, the involvement of β-endorphin in the often reported lack of pain perception on the battlefield, or following severe accidents has been suggested. In this respect β-endorphin has been compared to adrenaline, which not only acts as a neurotransmitter but also plays an essential role in the fight and flight reaction (25). Similarly, β-endorphin could mediate neuronal changes of a more lasting nature, for example as a neuromodulator or by affecting neuro-endocrine function, as well as play an important function in pain regulation during severe stress. The simultaneous release of ACTH and β-endorphin from their common 31K precursor molecule and possibly adrenal medullary discharge of catecholamines by adrenal opioid peptides (14,15) could be in accordance with such a dual action.

Which then are the receptors that mediate these multiple β-endorphin effects ? β-Endorphin has about equal affinity for μ and δ receptors and thus appears less specific than enkephalin. This is in concert with the observed multiple actions of β-endorphin. The affinity of β-endorphin for the morphine (μ) receptor is comparable to that of morphine and higher than that of enkephalins. The affinity of β-endorphin for the enkephalin (δ) receptor is lower than that of enkephalin, but considerably higher than the affinity of morphine for this δ receptor. Shortening of the peptide chain of β-endorphin reduces its potency for both receptors. Interaction with either μ or δ receptors appears sufficient to initiate β-endorphin induced analgesia. For the interaction with CNS μ receptor the C-terminal segments of β-endorphin are essential. Removal of the N-terminal (enkephalin) sequence of β-endorphin gives rise to C-terminal fragments like β-LPH 66-91 that can inhibit β-endorphin or morphine induced analgesia. It has been speculated that such inhibitory peptides exist in the brain, playing a physiological role in the regulation of endorphin action (41). The involvement of δ receptors in analgesia is also apparent from studies with metkephamid, a systemically active analgesic enkephalin analogue that preferentially interacts with δ receptors (42). The existence of separate β-endorphin "receptors" in the CNS has been demonstrated only very recently (43,44,45,46). Polypeptides often exhibit high non-receptor binding and different approaches have been developed to prevent this. Another important reason for the delay of direct binding studies has been a lack of availability of radioactively labeled β-endorphin. Morphine and the enkephalins possess low affinities for these specific β-endorphin binding sites. Shortening of the polypeptide chain of β-endorphin reduces its affinity for β-endorphin receptor sites. In addition to the enkephalin pentapeptide sequence, the C-terminal region of β-endorphin appears to be important in the interaction of β-endorphin with the β-endorphin receptor. Besides differences in affinity profiles, the three postulated opioid receptors also exhibit qualitative as well as quantitative differences in their sensitivity towards monovalent (Na^+) and divalent (Mn^{++}) cations and guanosine triphosphate (GTP). On the other hand, the three binding sites seem to share a common structural unit recognized by all three representative opioids, albeit with different affinities. It is as yet unknown if the altered sodium permeability and the GTP associated - and by divalent cations regulated - reduction of adenylate cyclase activity in synaptic actions of opioids are related or independent second messengers, communicating different kinds of information to the cell.

Finally, a range of different types of compounds appear to interact with opioid receptors to yield a pharmacological response. For example, other fragments of the 31 K precursor molecule - ACTH and MSH like peptides - have been shown to possess affinity for opioid receptors and to exhibit agonistic and antagonistic like actions (47,48). However, it is too early to speculate on the significance of such compounds.

6. CONCLUSION

There is good evidence for the existence of multiple opioid receptor sites in the CNS. These separate receptor systems, however, appear to share a common structural unit that is recognized by morphine, enkephalin and β-endorphin. This apparent lack of specificity and the supposed participation of opioids in modulating various neuronal pathways explain their multiple effects. These properties will hamper the development of new and better opioid analgesics for therapeutic use. On the other hand, the outlook appears bright in the light of the tremendous progress made since 1975 and the great potential of numerous candidates. The opioid receptors play a critical role in the developments and the recent succesful solubilization of an active opioid receptor (49,50) provides the basis for its further purifica-tion and characterization and hence for insight in its interaction with opioids.

REFERENCES

1. Kangawa K, Matsuo H, Igarashi M: α-Neo-endorphin: a "big" leu-enkephalin with potent opiate activity from porcine hypothalami. Biochem Biophys Res Commun 86: 153-160, 1979.
2. Goldstein A, Tachibana S, Lowney LI, Hunkapiller M, Hood L: Dynorphin-(1-13), an extraordinarily potent opioid peptide. Proc Natl Acad Sci USA 76: 6666-6670, 1979.
3. Goldstein A, Ghazarossian VE: Immunoreactive dynorphin in pituitary and brain. Proc Natl Acad Sci USA 77: 6207-6210, 1980.
4. Minamino N, Kangawa K, Fukuda A, Matsuo H, Iagarashi M: A new opioid octapeptide related to dynorphin from porcine hypothalamus. Biochem Biophys Res Commun 95: 1475-1481, 1980.
5. Kangawa K, Mizuno K, Minamino N, Matsuo H: Radioimmunoassay for detecting Pro-Leu-enkephalins in tissue extracts: purification and identification of [Arg6]-Leu-enkephalin in porcine pituitary. Biochem Biophys Res Commun 95: 1467-1474, 1980.
6. Kimura S, Lewis RV, Stern AS, Rossier J, Stein S, Udenfriend S: Probable precursors of [Leu]enkephalin and [Met]enkephalin in adrenal medulla: peptides of 3-5 kilodaltons. Proc Natl Acad Sci USA 77: 1681-1685, 1980.
7. Yang H-YT, Hexum T, Costa E: Opioid peptides in adrenal gland. Life Sci 27: 1119-1125, 1980.
8. Mizuno K, Minamino N, Kangawa K, Matsuo H: A new endogenous opioid peptide from bovine adrenal medulla: isolation and amino acid sequence of a dodecapeptide (BAM-12P). Biochem Biophys Res Commun 95: 1482-1488, 1980.
9. Mizuno K, Minamino N, Kangawa K, Matsuo H: A new family of endogenous "big" Met-enkephalins from bovine adrenal medulla: purification and structure of docosa- (BAM-22P) and eicosapeptide (BAM-20P) with very potent opiate activity. Biochem Biophys Res Commun 97: 1283-1290, 1980.
10. Stern AS, Lewis RV, Kimura S, Rossier J, Gerber LD, Brink L, Stein S, Udenfriend S: Isolation of the opioid heptapeptide Met-enkephalin-[Arg6,Phe7] from bovine adrenal medullary granules and striatum. Proc Natl Acad Sci USA 76: 6680-6683, 1979.
11. Huang W-Y, Chang RCC, Kastin AJ, Coy DH, Schally AV: Isolation and structure of pro-methionine-enkephalin: potential enkephalin precursor from porcine hypothalamus. Proc Natl Acad Sci USA 76: 6177-6180, 1979.
12. Takagi H, Shiomi H, Ueda H, Amano H: Morphine-like analgesia by a new dipeptide, L-Tyrosyl-L-Arginine (kyotorphin) and its analogue. Eur J Pharmacol 55: 109-111, 1979.
13. Takagi H, Shiomi H, Ueda H, Amano H: A novel analgesic dipeptide from bovine brain is a possible Met-enkephalin releaser. Nature 282: 410-412, 1979.
14. Slotkin TA, Burwell B, Lau C: An intracellular opiate receptor. Life Sci 27: 1975-1978, 1980.
15. Saria A, Wilson SP, Molnar A, Viveros OH, Lembeck F: Substance P and opiate-like peptides in human adrenal medulla. Neurosci Lett 20: 195-200, 1980.
16. Adler MW: Opioid peptides. Life Sci 26: 497-510, 1980.
17. Houghten RA, Swann RW, Li CH: β-Endorphin: stability, clearance behavior, and entry into the central nervous system after intravenous injection of the tritiated peptide in rats and rabbits. Proc Natl Acad Sci USA 77: 4588-4591, 1980.
18. Foley KM, Kourides IA, Inturrisi CE, Kaiko RF, Zaroulis CG, Posner JB, Houde RW, Li CH: β-Endorphin: analgesic and hormonal effects in humans. Proc Natl Acad Sci USA 76: 5377-5381, 1979.

19. Merin M, Höllt V, Przewlocki R, Herz A: Low permeation of systemically administered human β-endorphin into rabbit brain measured by radio-immunoassays differentiating human and rabbit β-endorphin. Life Sci 27: 281-289, 1980.

20. Snyder SH: Brain peptides as neurotransmitters. Science 209: 976-983, 1980.

21. Audigier Y, Mazarguil H, Gout R, Cros J: Structure-activity relation-ships of enkephalin analogs at opiate and enkephalin receptors: correlation with analgesia. Eur J Pharmacol 63: 35-46, 1980.

22. Martin WR, Eades CG, Thompson JA, Huppler RE, Gilbert PE: The effects of morphine- and nalorphine-like drugs in the nondependent and morphine-dependent chronic spinal dog. J Pharmacol Exp Ther 197: 517-532, 1976.

23. Wüster M, Schulz R, Herz A: The direction of opioid agonists towards μ-, δ- and ε-receptors in the vas deferens of the mouse and the rat. Life Sci 27: 163-170, 1980.

24. Chang K-J, Hazum E, Cuatrecasas P: Multiple opiate receptors. Trends Neurosci 3: 160-162, 1980.

25. Lord JAH, Waterfield AA, Hughes J, Kosterlitz HW: Endogenous opioid peptides: multiple agonists and receptors. Nature 267: 495-499, 1977.

26. Pasternak GW, Childers SR, Snyder SH: Opiate analgesia: evidence for mediation by a subpopulation of opiate receptors. Science 208: 514-516, 1980.

27. Chang K-J, Hazum E, Cuatrecasas P: Possible role of distinct morphine and enkephalin receptors in mediating actions of benzomorphan drugs (putative κ and σ agonists). Proc Natl Acad Sci USA 77: 4469-4473, 1980.

28. Feinberg AP, Creese I, Snyder SH: The opiate receptor: a model explaining structure-activity relationships of opiate agonists and antagonists. Proc Natl Acad Sci USA 73: 4215-4219, 1976.

29. Smith GD, Griffin JF: Conformation of [Leu^5]enkephalin from X-ray diffraction:features important for recognition at opiate receptor. Science 199: 1214-1216, 1978.

30. Gorin FA, Marshall GR: Proposal for the biologically active conformation of opiates and enkephalin. Proc Natl Acad Sci USA 74: 5179-5183, 1977.

31. Childers SR, Creese I, Snowman AM, Snyder SH: Opiate receptor binding affected differentially by opiates and opioid peptides. Eur J Pharmacol 55: 11-18, 1979.

32. Roques BP, Gacel G, Fournie-Zaluski M-C, Senault B, Lecomte J-M: Demonstration of the crucial role of the phenylalanine moiety in enkephalin analogues for differential recognition of the μ- and δ-receptors. Eur J Pharmacol 60: 109-110, 1979.

33. Wüster, M, Schulz R, Herz A: Opiate activity and receptor selectivity of dynorphin$_{1-13}$ and related peptides. Neurosci Lett 20: 79-83, 1980.

34. Herman BH, Leslie F, Goldstein A: Behavioral effects and in vivo degradation of intraventricularly administered dynorphin-(1-13) and D-Ala^2-dynorphin-(1-11) in rats. Life Sci 27: 883-892, 1980.

35. Inturrisi CE, Umans JG, Wolff D, Stern AS, Lewis RV, Stein S, Udenfriend S: Analgesic activity of the naturally occurring heptapeptide [Met]enkephalin-Arg^6-Phe^7. Proc Natl Acad Sci USA 77: 5512-5514, 1980.

36. Gintzler AR: Endorphin-mediated increases in pain threshold during pregnancy. Science 210: 193-195, 1980.

37. Fletcher JE, Hill RG, Thomas TA: β-Endorphin and parturition. Br J Pharmacol 70: 159P-160P, 1980.

38. Akil H, Watson SJ, Levy RM, Barchas JD: β-Endorphin and other 31 K fragments: pituitary and brain systems. In: Characteristics and function of opioids, van Ree JM, Terenius L (eds), Amsterdam, Elsevier/North-Holland Biomedical Press, 1978, p 123-134.

39. Clement-Jones V, Tomlin S, Rees LH, McLoughlin L, Besser GM, Wen HL: Increased β-endorphin but not Met-enkephalin levels in human cerebro-spinal fluid after acupuncture for recurrent pain. Lancet II: 946-949, 1980.

40. Abbate D, Santamaria A, Brambilla A, Panerai AE, Di Giulio AM: β-Endorphin and electroacupuncture. Lancet II: 1309, 1980.

41. Lee NM, Friedman HJ, Leybin L, Cho TM, Loh HH, Li CH: Peptide inhibitor of morphine- and β-endorphin-induced analgesia. Proc Natl Acad Sci USA 77: 5525-5526, 1980.

42. Frederickson RCA, Smithwick EL, Shuman R, Bemis KG: Metkephamid, a systemically active analog of Methionine enkephalin with potent opioid δ-receptor activity. Science 211: 603-605, 1981.

43. Akil H, Hewlett WA, Barchas JD, Li CH: Binding of ^{3}H-β-endorphin to rat brain membranes: characterization of opiate properties and inter-action with ACTH. Eur J Pharmacol 64: 1-8, 1980.

44. Ferrara P, Houghten R, Li CH: β-Endorphin: characteristics of binding sites in the rat brain. Biochem Biophys Res Commun 89: 786-792, 1979.

45. Ferrara P, Li CH: β-Endorphin: characteristics of binding sites in rabbit spinal cord. Proc Natl Acad Sci USA 77: 5746-5748, 1980.

46. Law P-Y, Loh HH, Li CH: Properties and localization of β-endorphin receptor in rat brain. Proc Natl Acad Sci USA 76: 5455-5459, 1979.

47. Walker JM, Akil H, Watson SJ: Evidence for homologous actions of pro-opiocortin products. Science 210: 1247-1249, 1980.

48. van Ree JM, Bohus B, Csontos KM, Gispen WH, Greven HM, Nijkamp FP, Opmeer FA, de Rotte AA, van Wimersma Greidanus Tj B, Witter A, de Wied D: Behavioral profile of γ-MSH: relationship with ACTH and β-endorphin action. Life Sci, in press.

49. Bidlack JM, Abood LG: Solubilization of the opiate receptor. Life Sci 27: 331-340, 1980.

50. Rüegg UT, Hiller JM, Simon EJ: Solubilization of an active opiate receptor from Bufo marinus. Eur J Pharmacol 64: 367-368, 1980.

FACTORS IN PHARMACOKINETICS OF ANALGESICS

W.Soudijn,
Department of Pharmaceutical Chemistry,
University of Amsterdam, The Netherlands.

Important parameters in analgesia are the dose of the narcotic
analgesic to be used, the onset of action and the duration
of action. These parameters are interrelated - that is - the
higher the doses, the quicker the onset of action and the
longer the duration of action.
In contrast to what is usually thought, the activity of the
drug - that is - its capability to interact efficiently with
its receptor resulting in a biological response, does not
necessarily correlate with the dose that has to be given to
evoke the required effect.

C O M P O U N D	I C $_{50}$ (nM.)	n	R E L A T I V E AFFINITY *
Etonitazene	.110	2	31
Fentanyl	1.14	5	3.0
Dihydromorphine	1.44	3	2.3
Naloxone	1.48	3	2.3
Dextromoramide	2.20	2	1.5
Morphine	3.37	4	1.0
dl-Methadone	3.52	3	.96
Codeine	385	3	.0088
Levomoramide	5140	2	.00066
(+)-Benzetimide (dexetimide)	20800	3	.00016
(-)-Benzetimide (levetimide)	26700	3	.00013

* morphine = 1.0

From Table 1 (dihydromorphine should of course read
dihydromorphine) showing the receptor affinity of several
narcotic- and some non-narcotic drugs some of which are

structurally related to fentanyl, can be seen that an anti-
tussive non-narcotic drug like levomoramide (the levo-isomer
of the narcotic drug dextromoramide), the new antiarrythmic
drug lorcaïnide, the potent anticholinergic drug d-benzetimide
or dexetimide and its inactive isomer l-benzetimide have virtually no affinity for the receptor for fentanyl.
This means that in this experiment, we are dealing with a
receptor that is specific for opiates.
The affinity of fentanyl for the opiate receptor is 3 times
higher than that of morphine but the analgetic dose of fentanyl
is about 60 times lower than that of morphine. That means that
fentanyl is much more potent than its receptor affinity fore-
tells. Codeïne has an affinity which is a hundred times less
than that of morphine but codeïne still has an appreciable
analgesic effect.
Not shown are the antidiarrheal drugs diphenoxylate and lope-
ramide which owe their effect to interaction with opiate receptors in the intestinal wall. They have an affinity for the
isolated receptor from the central nervous system comparable
to that of morphine. However, they are devoid of analgesic -
or any other central activity.
For a drug to have, an analgesic activity, the ability to
interact with the opiate receptor is evidently not sufficient.
It has to be able to reach the receptors in the central nervous system in a sufficient quantity by passing the blood-
brain barrier.
It is evident that the antidiarrheals cannot penetrate the
blood-brain barrier, at least not in amounts large enough to
build up a large enough concentration at the receptor site.
Fentanyl is clinically more active than morphine because it
penetrates the blood-brain barrier much easier than morphine.
That is because fentanyl is more lipophylic than morphine
which is rather hydrophilic and which passes the barrier with
difficulty. On the other hand, once morphine has penetrated
the blood-brain barrier it will stay longer in the brain than

fentanyl because in order to get out, it again has to cross
certain lipid barriers. From these considerations alone, we
may tentatively conclude that fentanyl will have a quicker
onset and a shorter duration of action than morphine .
The hydrophylicity of morphine stems from the presence of
two hydroxy groups. (Table 2)

STRUCTURE	R (name)	IC_{50}(nM)	RELATIVE AFFINITY
	H (3-deoxymorphine)	--	--
	OH (morphine)	3.37	1.0
	OCH$_3$ (codeine)	385	.0088
	H (Ph 6013)	74.3	.045
	OH (Ph 2157)	.98	3.4
	OCH$_3$ (Ph 2438)	49.7	.068

In codeïne the phenolic hydroxy group of morphine has been
substituted by an methoxy group (OCH$_3$) thereby enhancing its
lipophylicity and capability of crossing the blood-brain
barrier, better than morphine, so that a high concentration
may be reached at the receptor level. As far as I know there
are no data on the penetration of codeïne in the brain but I
may easily be mistaken.
There is however another factor which may also explain the
analgesic activity of codeïne and that is the possibility of
biotransformation of some codeine into morphine by demethy-
lation.
In the group of the morphines, the morphinans (not shown,
prototype levorphanol) and the benzomorphans, the presence
of an hydroxy group on the aromatic ring is an absolute requirement for a good fit on the receptor and analgesic acti-

vity as can be seen from table 2. The receptor affinity of
benzomorphan Ph2157 is comparable to that of fentanyl while
the derivates without an hydroxy group or with a methoxy
group show a rather poor affinity. The analgesic activity in
vivo of Ph2157 is about 10 times less than that of fentanyl,
again as a result from its lower lipophylicity.

Often it is assumed that factors like plasma proteïnbinding
and ionization of the drug are important factors governing
tissue penetration and thus onset of action, because only the
free, uncharged drug is able, to penetrate the membrane barriers,
and in cases of high plasma proteïnbinding and a large fraction of the drug in the charged state there is very little
free drug travelling around with the blood.
Most analgesics used in clinical practice are basic amines
with pk_a values ranging from 7.9 to 9.2 which means that they
are present in the blood in the charged form for 70 to 90%.
Moreover they are bound to plasma proteïns to a considerable
extent let us say from 70% and over. Take for instance a drug
like fentanyl, it is bound for about 70-80% to plasma proteïn
and the nonbound fraction in the plasma water is for 90% in
the charged state. This leaves us with very very little of
uncharged distributable drug.
Now we all know what happens, when we inject fentanyl in man
let's say in a dose of 6 µg/kg intra venously (Fig.1).Within 5 minutes after the injection, 95% of the fentanyl has left the
plasma and pharmacological effects may already be noted.
Transfer of the drug from the plasma to the extracellular
interstitial fluid would only account for a 50% lowering of
the plasma concentration. So tissue penetration must be the
cause of the drastic lowering of the fentanyl plasmalevel as
can be seen in Fig.2 where the results are shown of the tissue
distribution of fentanyl in the rabbit after administration
of 20 µg per kg intra venously. Already half a minute after
the injection several tissuelevels especially in tissues
with a high blood flow relative to their mass like lung,

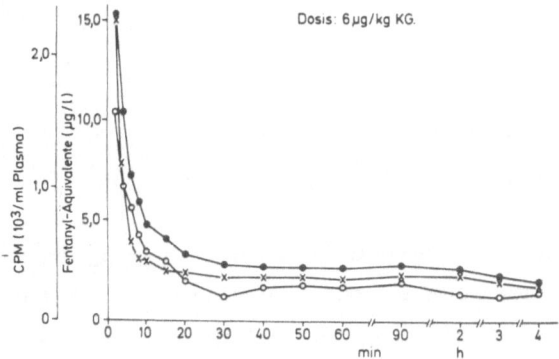

Fig.1.
H.Schauer and E.Jenny, In W.F.Henschel, Neue
Klinische Aspekte der Neuroleptanalgesie.
Schattauer Verlag 1970.

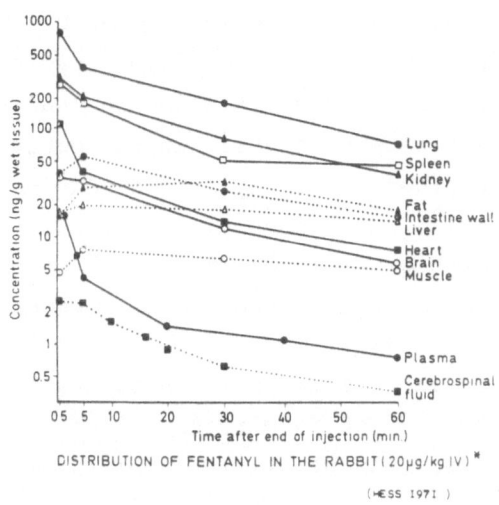

Fig.2.
R.Hess et al, J.Pharmacol. Exp. Ther.192 677
(1971).

kidney, heart and brain, are very much higher than the plasma
fentanyllevel. The solution to this seeming contradiction is
simple but very often overlooked, with the result that the
effect of plasma proteïnbinding and presence of the charged
state is very often overrated.

Generally these phenomena are not limiting factors for the
tissue distribution of narcotic drugs.

$$BOUNDDRUG \rightleftharpoons FREEDRUG$$

$$CHARGED\ DRUG \rightleftharpoons UNCHARGED\ DRUG$$

Plasmaproteïnbinding and charged state are _dynamic_ equilibrium
phenomena, that is, as soon as the concentration of the free
drug in the plasma is declining because of tissue penetration
of the free drug, the equilibrium is disturbed and the system
tries to re-establish the original state by shifting the equi-
libria to the right that is by supplying more free drug, which
is immediately taken up by the tissues. The overall result
is a rapid decline in plasma drug levels. Organs with a high
bloodflow and a large capillary bed providing an enormous
surface for penetration will pick up the drug very rapidly.
I am aware of the fact that changes in blood pH leading to alkalosis of acidosis, and causing a shift in the equilibrium
charged state $\leftrightarrow$ uncharged state may have a considerable
effect on pharmacokinetics and tissue distribution of the
drug. These effects may however rather be caused by changes
in the state of the membranes and thus in their permeability
than in changes of the equilibrium.
There may however be small effects as was shown by Brown,
Pleuvry and Kay who studied the respiratory effects of a new
very shortacting analgesic Alfentanyl in rabbits.
Alfentanyl is a close relative-structurally and pharmacologically speaking- of fentanyl. It is about 4 times less potent than fentanyl and has a much shorter duration of action.
In rats at 4 times the minimal ED_{50} is has a duration of analgesic actions of only 18 minutes while fentanyl has a duration of action of 54 minutes at 4 x its minimal ED_{50}.
Alfentanyl is only for 10% ionized (charged) in the plasma
while fentanyl is ionized for 90%. We assume that the plasma
proteïnbinding of both compounds is about the same, as data
is not available yet.

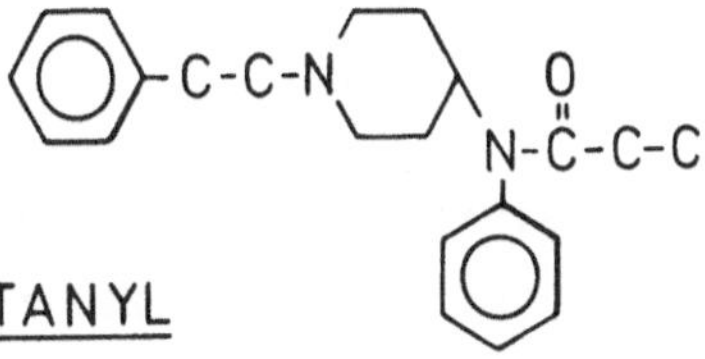

RATS

	ED_{50}min mg/kg	Duration of action $4 \times ED_{50}$min

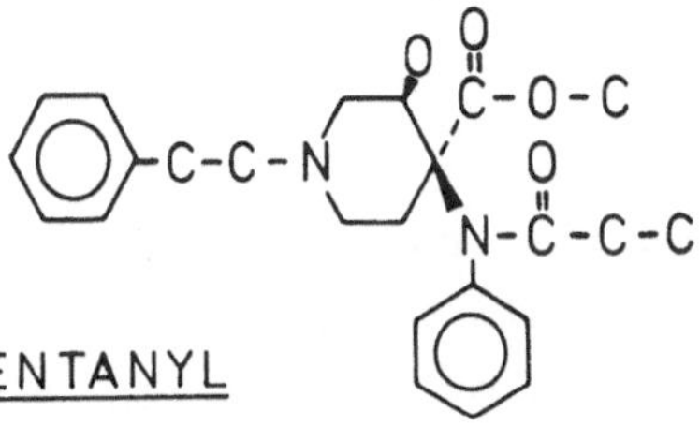

FENTANYL

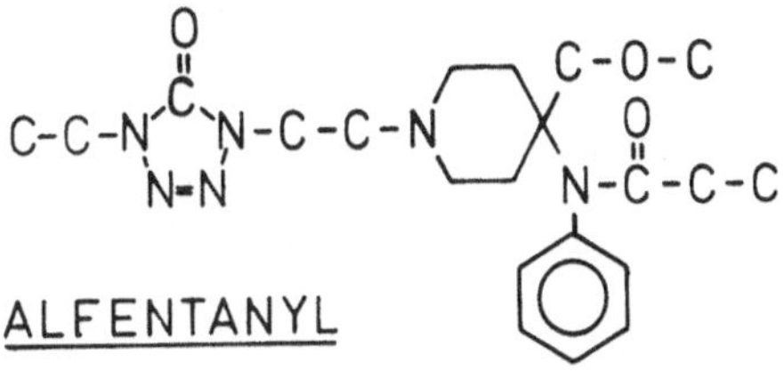

0.011   54 min.

ALFENTANYL

0.043   18 min.

LOFENTANYL

0.00059   >12 hours

Back to the rabbits: The peak effect of depression of respiratory frequency after intravenous injection 10 µg/kg of alfentanyl occurred at 3 minutes and the effect was nearly over at 15 minutes after the injection. Fentanyl gave a maximal depression at 5 minutes, a statistically significant but small and unimportant difference, but the effect lasted much longer. Twenty minutes after the injection there was still a marked depression.

Repeated doses of fentanyl had a cumulative effect on depression of respiratory frequency, while repeated doses of alfentanyl did not show a cumulative effect at all.

The potency of alfentanyl in man is about 1/3 of that of fentanyl and the duration of action is also about 1/3 of that
of fentanyl.

The duration of action

The duration of action of narcotic analgesics depends obviously on the rate of elimination of the drug and its pharmacologically active metabolites - if there are any - from
the target tissue, the central nervous system. The rate of
elimination depends on the rate of biotransformation of the
drug mainly in the liver although hydrolysis and glucuroni-
dation can also effectively occur in the gut wall and on
the amount that can be stored in other tissues like fat
tissue and skeletal muscle.

The storage capacity of the individual skeletal muscle may
be very small and the rate of uptake may be somewhat lower
than in tissues like brain, liver, kidney and heart, but
because of its large mass the accumalation can be considerable.

Hug calculated that 5 minutes after injection 55% of the
dose may be stored in skeletal muscle from which it is slow-
ly released in the course of time. This may be the cause of
the rather long and similar halflives of elimination of drugs
like morphine, pethidine (meperidine) fentanyl and pentazo-
cine of about 3-3,5 hours.

As most of the narcotic analgesics are fairly lipophylic
drugs, the portion of the drug that is excreted unchanged,
is generally rather small, so all these drugs are extensively metabolized into highly hydrophilic compounds before they
can be excreted. Higher doses lead to higher plasmalevels of
the drug for a longer period of time as Murphy and Hug showed
when they injected fentanyl at a dose of 10 μg/kg or a dose
of 100 μg/kg in dogs (Fig.3). It is generally assumed that
the exchange of narcotic analgesics between plasma and brain
happens, according to an open compartment model, that is the

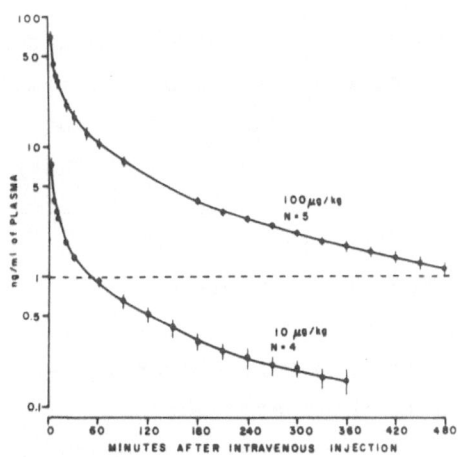

Fig.3.
Murphy M.R. et al
Anesthesiology 50 13 (1979).

brain concentration in the brain is in dynamic equilibrium
with the concentration in the plasma. I personally doubt
whether this is also true for a very long acting drug like
lofentanyl (more than 12 hours at 4 times the minimal ED_{50}
in rats), which is probably strongly bound in the receptor-
compartment of the central nervous system, but when there is
a free exchange between narcotic in the brain and in the
plasma, than it is obvious that higher plasma levels during
a longer period will lead to a more intense analgesic effect
and respiratory depression of longer duration.
The same holds true for repeated injections of most narcotic
analgesics with the exception probably of alfentanyl as
shown in the experiments of Brown et al.
The phenomenon can be explained in several ways; It is possible that the stores in skeletal muscle are becoming more
or less saturated. It is also possible that the metabolizing
enzymes in the liver become saturated or become inhibited
by the metabolites they are producing. This is a common

phenomenon in enzymology. It is also conceivable that both processes are operating at the same time.

The short duration of action of a drug like alfentanyl might be explained by the fact that it has a 5-10 times lower affinity for the opiate receptor than fentanyl sufentanyl and lofentanyl, the latter having a very high affinity and that the drug is extensively and very rapidly metabolized following only partly the same metabolic pathways as fentanyl, giving rise to more and different metabolites.

In this way the chances that all the metabolizing enzymes are blocked at the same time are very slight indeed. I would now like to discuss briefly the pharmacokinetic problem, - if that's what it is - of the delayed or biphasic respiratory depression as is reported to occur sometimes, even after small doses of fentanyl.

Sometimes a sudden rise in the plasma fentanyl level is seen in some but not in all the patients. Sometimes the rise occurs in the redistribution phase as shown in the work of Sebel and Bovill and Stoeckel, sometimes the rise occurs in the elimination phase. MacQuay found in 60% of patients within 45 minutes of the end of surgery peaks in the plasma curve of fentanyl. Stoeckel et al on the basis of their own experiments concluded that this was due to excretion of fentanyl in the stomach and re-uptake after transport from the stomach to the small intestine into the circulation (In man 16% of the administered dose of fentanyl was found in the stomachwall 10 minutes after the injection). This phenomenon of excretion and re-uptake should explain the occurrence of delayed respiratory depression. I find this explanation difficult to accept, because:

Firstly transportation along the gastro intestinal tract in the presence of an narcotic analgesic must be minimal.

Secondly when fentanyl is absorbed from the intestine, it has to pass the liver were it is for the greater part metabolized. It is well known from pharmacology that the potency of fentanyl, when orally given is at least 10 times less than

when given intravenously, just because of this very large
first-pass effect. If the secondary respiratory depression
correlates with the sudden rise in plasma level of fentanyl,
the source of the fentanyldelivery is to be sought elsewhere
for instance in the skeletal muscle. The why and how however,
is still not clear at all, at least not to me.

In the recovery period there is of course a variation in the
intensity of stimuli for the patient. As soon as the patient
is left alone or at least not talked too, the central neuronal activity diminishes or at least changes. This can make
the opiate receptor more sensitive to residual fentanyl for
instance by a mechanism of competition between fentanyl and
endogenous inhibitors of the opiate receptor or by a change
in the micro-environment of the opiate receptor as it is well
known that these receptors are sensitive to e.g. sodium ions.
In the presence of sodium ions the affinity of narcotic agonists for the receptor is much less than in the absence of
sodium ions, while the affinity of pure antagonists like naloxone for instance remains the same. Lowering of the sodium
concentration in the direct environment of the receptor can
make this receptor more sensitive to fentanyl. It would be
very interesting to know whether this phenomenon of delayed
respiratory depression also occurs when other narcotic analgesics like pethidine, morphine, or levorphanol are used,
any way narcotics with another chemical structure than fentanyl.

There exist of course in patients a host of factors influencing the duration of action or rather the pharmacokinetics
of narcotic drugs.

There is the influence of age. In the newborn a 7 fold increase in the elimination halflife of pethidine was found and
the excretion with the urine was delayed. Elderly patients
show a 2 fold increase in plasmaconcentration of pethidine
compared to younger patients after intramuscular injection.
This increase is due to a decrease in the distribution vo-

lume which means that the binding of pethidine to tissue components and probably to certain tissue compartments like for instance skeletal muscle has decreased.

Diseases may also alter the pharmacokinetics of drugs.

In livercirrhosis or acute hepatitis the elimination halflife of pethidine is more than doubled because the plasma clearance through the uptake and biotransformation in the liver is impaired.

Corall reported in 1980 that the elimination halflife of fentanyl is not significantly prolonged in patients with severe chronic liver disease.

In patients with renal failure (if not on haemodialysis) a prolonged action of narcotic analgesics is to be expected. Hess showed in anephric rabbits a prolongation of the elimination halflife of fentanyl and, a higher plasma concentration of the drug. It is feasible that through accumulation of fentanyl metabolites, the rate of biotransformation of fentanyl has slowed down because of endproduct inhibition of the metabolizing enzymes. In patients a prolonged action is to be expected not only from a prolonged halflife of the unchanged analgesic but also from a build-up in the concentration of metabolites with potential analgesic activity.

The major metabolites of fentanyl are devoid of analgesic activity but not all the metabolites are known yet. There is a possibility that one of the aromatic rings is hydroxylated in the paraposition (OH group opposite to the other substituent groups of the phenyl rings). We synthesized these products and determined their affinity to the opiate receptor in vitro. We found that parahydroxylation of the phenyl ring of the phenethyl group (phenyl ring on the left side of the structure) leads to a product with a low affinity - about 0,05 of that of fentanyl - while parahydroxylation of the anilinophenyl ring (ring at the right side) leads to a product with virtually the same affinity as fentanyl for the opiate receptor. It is not known yet, whether this product is indeed a biotransformationproduct of fentanyl.

REFERENCES

Bovill, J.G., Sebel, P.S., Brit.J.Anaesth. 1980, 52 795.

Brown, J.H., Pleuvry, B.J., Kay, B., Brit.J.Anaesth. 1980, 52 1101.

Corall, I.M., Moore, A.R., Strunin, L., Brit.J.Anaesth. 1980, 52 101.

McQuay, H.J., Moore, R.A., Paterson, G.M.C., Adams, A.P. Brit.J.Anaesth. 1979, 51 543.

Murphy, M.R., Olson, W.A., Hug, C.C., Anesthesiology 1979, 50 13.

Stoeckel, H., Hengstman, J.H., Schütter, J., Brit.J.Anaesth. 1979, 51 741.

THE PHYSIOLOGICAL BACKGROUND OF STRESS-FREE ANESTHESIA

T.H. STANLEY

The concept of stress-free anesthesia is, in fact, a relatively new idea. It was born as recently as February, 1978 at a Symposium in Belgium entitled "Stress-Free Anesthesia - Analgesia and Depression of Stress Responses".[1] At that Symposium, a number of papers were presented which suggested that if sufficiently high doses of fentanyl were administered intravenously, cardiovascular dynamics remain unchanged and increases in plasma cortisol, antidiuretic hormone, growth hormone, the catecholamines, glucose, lactate, and some of the sex hormones which occur normally with induction of anesthesia and initiation of surgery, could be attenuated or totally blocked.[2-5] There is little argument that stability of cardiovascular dynamics during induction of anesthesia and throughout surgery is a desirable end. Whether the same is also true of the normal stress responding hormones remains to be carefully documented.

Although blockade of stress responding hormones has been demonstrated for many years to be achievable with adequate levels of spinal and epidural anesthesia, this has never been the case in patients who have undergone general anesthesia. Thus, general anesthesia has usually been associated with stimulation of what could be very simply called "the stress response".[2] Recent studies have confirmed that large doses of fentanyl,[6] sufentanil (Stanley TH, unpublished data), alfentanil (Stanley TH, unpublished data) and morphine[7] can block normal stress responding hormones as well as the heightened sympathetic activity associated with profound surgical stimulation. Stanley and co-workers,[4,6-8] as well as Philbin et al, (unpublished data) have demonstrated that hemodynamic stability is usually associated with hormonal stability although the presence of one does not necessarily insure the other. While increases in heart rate, arterial blood pressure, myocardial contractility and peripheral vascular resistance are obviously dangerous in certain patients, i.e., patients with coronary artery disease, whether increases in plasma catecholamines and the other stress responding hormones are also disadvantageous to similar patients is unclear. It is possible that in certain patients an increase in some or more of these hormones may be desirable. For example, patients with severe mitral stenosis who have an impaired cardiac output and have marked increases in circulating epinephrine and norepinephrine preoperatively might, in fact, require such elevations in their plasma catecholamines to insure cardiovascular stability. A decrease in such catecholamine levels or no alteration of these hormones in response to painful stimulation may result in inadequate blood supply to muscles and other organs which have increased blood and oxygen needs. On the other hand, elevations in these catecholamines increase myocardial as well as other organ system oxygen requirements. Increases in oxygen requirements are disadvantageous to patients with ischemic cardiac disease. These patients suffer from a basic inability to supply blood and oxygen to their myocardium and any physiological condition which increases the requirements for oxygen delivery to this tissue has to be viewed as detrimental.

One of the exciting findings of studies involving the fentanyl series of narcotics has been their success as anesthetics in open heart and major vascular surgery and the interesting changes which have been observed during cardiopulmonary bypass.[6,8] When given in "anesthetic doses", doses that block cardiovascular responses to surgery, there is a decrease or no increase in plasma catecholamines, antidiuretic hormone, human growth hormone, and cortisol up until cardiopulmonary bypass. This absence of hormonal response does not, however, persist during bypass. Indeed, studies with fentanyl have indicated that there are marked rises in catecholamines and antidiuretic hormone during this physiologic state. Similar studies recently performed using sufentanil and alfentanil have shown that these newer narcotics block antidiuretic hormone increases during bypass and the post-bypass period but do not block increases in epinephrine and norepinephrine (de Lange S, Stanley TH, unpublished data). These recent data indicate that sufentanil in doses of approximately 14 ug/kg and alfentanil in doses of approximately 1-1.2 mg/kg are effective in blocking some of the stress responses of cardiopulmonary bypass but not all of them. Cardiopulmonary bypass is associated with many alterations in the circulatory system. In most centers, bypass is conducted with a non-pulsatile type of extracorporeal circuit and hemodilution. In

addition, hypothermia and a variety of other drugs are used during this
state. Exactly which of these many conditions is the principal cause of
the marked stress response associated with bypass is unknown. Indeed, as
during the pre-bypass period or anesthesia and surgery in general, it is
difficult to say whether blockade of such responses is advantageous or
disadvantageous. We simply do not know which direction we should point.
Still, the overall impression is that blockade of the stress response
would appear, from what we do know, to be a desirable action.

There are some data, and this is unpublished work, which suggests that
narcotizing patients in an Intensive Care Unit may be protective to those
who are hypermetabolic. Such narcotization is usually associated with an
unchanged cardiac output, a reduced heart rate and a decrease in total
body oxygen consumption and CO_2 production. Theoretically, these changes
may be advantageous in situations where a patient's circulation cannot
meet the overall metabolic demand. Such a situation would, of course,
exist in patients in septic shock. Data from our operating rooms indicate
that the use of large doses of fentanyl in patients in septic shock is
desirable because patients are able to withstand the stress of surgery
without alteration of cardiovascular dynamics.[9] In addition, the resuscitation and operative procedure can be accomplished without fear of cardiovascular or metabolic collapses secondary to anesthetic complications.
Further work is obviously needed in this area, as in the operating room,
under more controlled conditions, in order to substantiate or disprove
the benefit of narcotics as agents that block the surgical stress response. However, what information is available is exciting and suggestive
that we are at the beginning of a new era in anesthesiology and critical
care medicine.

REFERENCES

1. Wood C: Stress-Free Anaesthesia. Grune & Stratton, New York, 1978
2. Hall GM: Analgesia and the metabolic response to surgery. In Stress-
   Free Anaesthesia, Edited by Wood C, Grune & Stratton, New York, 1978,
   pp 19-22.
3. Florence A: Attenuation of stress and haemodynamic stability. In
   Stress-Free Anaesthesia, Edited by Wood C, Grune & Stratton, New York,
   1978, pp 23-24.
5. Ott E and Martin E: Stress in neurolept anaesthesia for patients
   with mitral valve disease. In Stress-Free Anaesthesia, Edited by
   Wood C, Grune & Stratton, New York, 1978, pp 27-32
6. Stanley TH, Berman L, Green O, Robertson DH: Plasma catecholamine
   and cortisol responses, Anesthesiology 53:250-253, 1980.

7. Stanley TH, Isern-Amaral J, Lathrop GD: The effects of morphine anes-
    thesia on urine norepinephrine during and after coronary artery sur-
    gery. Can Anaesth Soc J 22:478-485, 1975.
8. Stanley TH, Philbin DM, Coggins CH: Fentanyl-oxygen anesthesia for
    coronary artery surgery: cardiovascular and antidiuretic hormone
    responses. Canad Anaesth Soc J 26:168-172, 1979.
9. Stanley TH, Reddy P: Fentanyl-oxygen anesthesia in septic shock.
    Anesthesiology 51:S100, 1979.

NEW DEVELOPMENTS IN THE USE OF HIGH DOSE NARCOTIC TECHNIQUES FOR
CORONARY ARTERY SURGERY.

S. de LANGE.

Introduction

The use of Fentanyl as a complete narcotic anaesthetic agent for open heart
surgery has become an established technique. It can provide a stable
haemodynamic background for cardiac surgery. In addition, fentanyl in high
doses appears to control some of the endocrine and metabolic responses to
surgery[1,4,5].

High dose Fentanyl anaesthesia does have some disadvantages: its onset of
action is slow which results in a long induction time, induction of
anaesthesia is associated with a moderate incidence of muscle rigidity[6,7]
and at times of maximal surgical stress haemodynamic breakthrough does
sometimes occur[8]. Once this breakthrough is established it may be difficult to control even with further large doses of Fentanyl. These high
doses may then result in an unduly prolonged recovery and extubation
time[2,9]. For the past eighteen months at the University clinic of Leiden,
we have been examining high dose narcotic techniques for coronary artery
bypass grafting operations. Our aim was to shorten the induction time yet
neither increase the incidence of rigidity nor decrease cardiovascular
stability at this time. We also wanted to provide stress free anaesthesia.
In coronary artery disease the oxygenation of the myocardium is already
in jeopardy, increasing the rate pressure product and hereby the oxygen
requirements could lead to serious sequelae.

Firstly we studied Fentanyl in order to try and improve its performance
as a "stress free" narcotic anaesthetic agent. Then we compared Fentanyl
with two new synthetic morphomimetics, Alfentanil and Sufentanil used as
sole anaesthetic agents for coronary artery surgery. We examined the cardiovascular parameters of surgical stress in this report, the endocrine
and metabolic profiles are reported elsewhere.

FENTANYL

Standard experimental technique

Our patients received an oral Lorazepam premedication (0.08 mg/kg)
2 hours before arriving in the operating room. Half an hour before this
they had an intramuscular injection of 0.5 mg Atropine. In the operating
room ECG recording was established and percutaneous radial artery cannu-
lation performed. After the necessary intravenous cannulae had been introduced, a Swan Ganz catheter (7 French IL) was introduced via a vein in
the upper extremity. The patient was allowed to settle and control measurements made including thermodilution cardiac output. After preoxygenation
(2 minutes)and precurarisation with pancuronium (0.02 mg/kg) Fentanyl was
injected intravenously at the rate of 400 μg/minute until the patient
was unconscious.

In the half hour between induction and incision we infused twice the induction dose of Fentanyl which resulted in an average dose by incision of
60 μg/kg. We aimed at a dose of this magnitude since at this level the
EEG exhibits a large amplitude slow wave activity associated with deep
sleep (Personal communication J. Bovill M.D.). After induction the
patients were intubated after using succinylcholine as muscle relaxant
and then ventilated with 100% oxygen throughout the operation. Twenty
minutes after induction pancuronium 0.08 mg/kg was given for muscle relaxation. Once surgery had commenced we gave a bolus doses of Fentanyl
(250 μg/bolus) and repeated this dose up to three times if necessary so
that our systolic blood pressure would not exceed 15% of our preoperative
control level.

Measurements (For all the experimental techniques)

1. Dose and time to unconsciousness.
2. Incidence of rigidity.
3. Cardiovascular dynamics (including cardiac output).
   At fixed times throughout the operation.
4. A rise of systolic blood pressure up to 20% or more of preoperative
   control values.
   Measurements were recorded throughout the procedure but especially at
   times of maximum surgical stress eg. sternotomy and maximal sternal
   spread.
5. Total dose of narcotic required.

6. The use of supplements.

  If the three bolus doses of narcotic failed to keep the systolic blood
  pressure rise to 20% of the control value then vasodilators were used.
  Phentolamine (1-3 mg) pre- and during bypass and sodium nitroprusside
  (0.5-2 μg/kg/min) after bypass. Before commencing nitroprusside however, nitrous oxide (25% to 50% oxygen) was administered.

7. The recovery time.

  The time that patients returned to consciousness and the time the patients were extubatable. (It is the policy of our surgeons and our ICU
  to ventilate these patients until the morning of the postoperative day).
  The patients had been kept sedated until this point but were then
  allowed to be ventilated throughout the night with further sedation or
  analgesics (usually half doses were sufficient, if at all necessary).
  The patients were not considered extubatable until they could fulfil
  several ventilatory tests without continuous verbal support after a
  two hour stable cardiovascular period[9].

Fentanyl high dose technique

Animal studies have shown that after intravenous lofentanil, narcosis and
rigidity occur when there is a 25% occupancy of the opiate receptors in
the cortex[10]. We extrapolated that in man it might be possible that a
stress response might occur if the cortical opiate receptors were not fully
occupied. Therefore, we decided to infuse four times the induction dose
by incision as compared to twice this dose with the standard technique. We
then continue the high initial dose technique in the same way as the standard technique.
We looked at two groups of 10 patients randomly selected and all about to
undergo coronary artery bypass grafting operation.

Results

Prebypass heart rate and cardiac output remained unchanged in both groups.
Post bypass cardiac output was not considered as a suitable parameter for
this study since it was frequently much increased probably due to diluti-
onal and other effects of cardio-pulmonary bypass.

FENTANYL REQUIREMENTS (µg/kg)

	Uncons.	Incis.	Bypass	End op.
F. STANDARD	27	60	99	117
F. HIGH	28	119	133	136

With the standard technique a further 65% of the incision dose was re-quired by bypass time; whereas with the high dose technique only a further approx 15% of the incision dose. Fentanyl had to be given throughout the procedure with the standard regime yet with the high dose technique, after bypass commenced, very little further Fentanyl was required.

RISE IN SBP 20% OR GREATER (%)

	Intub.	Incis.	Stern.	S. Spread
F. STANDARD	0	10	40	60
F. HIGH	0	0	10	10

About 50% of the standard group manifested cardiovascular breakthrough whereas only 10% of the high group reacted in this manner to peak surgi-cal stress.

PATIENTS REQUIRING SUPPLEMENTATION (%)

	Before CPB	CPB	After CPB	
	Phentolamine		N_2O	SNP
F. STANDARD	40	50	60	40
F. HIGH	10	0	20	10

Between 40 and 50% of the standard group required vasodilators for cardio-vascular stability. In the high group there was only a 10% incidence.

RECOVERY TIMES
(hours post op.)

	Conscious	Extubatable
F. STANDARD	2.2	4.6
F. HIGH	6.4	7.5 [x]

[x] Based on 3 patients extubatable within 10 hours.

The high group took 3 times as long to regain consciousness as the standard group. Only three of 10 patients in the high dose group were considered extubatable within the study period. Seven patients were not extubatable until after the postoperative study period of 10 hours. In fact, three of these seven patients could not be extubated until 24 hours postoperatively.

Fentanyl standard versus high dose technique.

Using the standard method of Fentanyl narcosis it was often necessary to use vasodilators and an anaesthetic supplement (N_2O) to maintain good cardiovascular stability.

The high dose technique afforded excellent cardiovascular stability with infrequent use of supplements. However recovery and extubation time were often unduly prolonged.

Alfentanil

Alfentanil is a short acting narcotic related to Fentanyl. It was introduced in 1976 and it has one third the duration of action and about one third the potency of Fentanyl[11].

Using this drug we considered it possible that we could achieve deep narcotic anaesthesia with stable cardiovascular dynamics yet reduce the recovery time.

Method

A group of 15 randomly chosen patients were selected. After identical preparations as for the two Fentanyl groups, the patients were induced after precurarisation with pancuronium (0.02 mg/kg) using Alfentanil at a rate of 3 mg per minute. After unconsciousness anaesthesia was maintained with 2.5 mg bolus doses repeated as necessary three times using the same parameters as with Fentanyl. It was not possible to limit our technique to giving twice or even four times the induction dose by incision time due to the evanescent action of the narcotic. After intubation (using succinylcholine as muscle relaxant) full curarisation was not given before 20 minutes had lapsed. By this time, during catheterisation and other preparatory procedures, level of consciousness could be assessed until a sufficient loading dose of the narcotic had been given to ensure unconsciousness.

Results

Again cardiac output and heart rate were stable with this technique pre-bypass.

INDUCTION TIME

F. STANDARD	4.9 mins
ALFENTANIL	1.25 mins (75 seconds)

Unconsciousness occurred three times faster than with the Fentanyl techniques described. We found that we could give Alfentanil relatively faster than Fentanyl (after a initial pilot study) yet the incidence of rigidity ($\pm$ 25%) was the same.

RISE IN SBP 20% OR GREATER (%)

	Intub.	Incis.	Stern.	S. Spread
F. STANDARD	0	10	40	60
ALFENTANIL	0	0	60	73

Comparing Alfentanil with the Fentanyl standard technique, indicated that incidence of haemodynamic stress response was similar.

PATIENTS REQUIRING SUPPLEMENTATION (%)

	Before CPB	CPB	After CPB	
		Phentolamine	N_2O	SNP
F. STANDARD	40	50	60	40
ALFENTANIL	0	27	47	33

The action of Alfentanil is so rapid (one circulation time) that although the stress response was exhibited as frequently as with Fentanyl, no supplements were required pre bypass.

Also, during bypass, and after bypass we could reduce the use of vasodilators and nitrous oxide with the alfentanil group.

RECOVERY TIMES
(hours post op.)

	Conscious	Extubatable
F. STANDARD	2.2	4.6
ALFENTANIL	1.4	4.1

Patients receiving Alfentanil were awake 33% faster than with Fentanyl. Although not indicated by the figures we found that the extubatable time was more definite and with less variation than with Fentanyl.

Alfentanil versus standard Fentanyl

1. There is a considerably shorter induction time (1/3) with Alfentanil yet with similar cardiovascular stability and with the same incidence of rigidity as with Fentanyl.
2. The recovery of consciousness is faster.
3. It needs to be given often and throughout the operation to maintain a good cardiovascular stability and anaesthetic level.
4. Alfentanil controls the haemodynamic stress response faster than Fentanyl; the stress response does not have time to establish itself and thus the use of vasodilators may be avoided or reduced.

Sufentanil

Introduced in 1974, Sufentanil has the same duration of action of Fentanyl yet 5-10 times its potency and a very large safety margin[11]. Increased potency may be associated with greater specificity for the receptors and could possibly result in even more stable anaesthesia than with other narcotics. With this in mind we evaluated the role of Sufentanil as a complete narcotic anaesthetic and compared it with a standard Fentanyl technique.

Methods

40 patients for coronary artery bypass grafting operations were randomly assigned Sufentanil or Fentanyl.

Premedication, preparations and monitoring were the same as with the standard technique described before with one exception:

All patients receiving β-adrenergic blockers received their usual morning oral dose with their oral premedication two hours pre-operatively. After pre-oxygenation and pre-curarisation (1.5 mg/75 kg) Sufentanil was injected at a rate of 300 µg/min. The induction dose was doubled by incision time. Then further 50 µg increments of Sufentanil were given and repeated three times if necessary to keep within our control levels as described before. If this regime failed to control the haemodynamic stress response vasodilators were used. Fentanyl narcosis was given according to the standard regime.

Results

1.

	INDUCTION		RIGIDITY (%)		
	Time (min)	None	Mild	Severe	Total
Fentanyl	4.6	78	16	5	21
Sufentanil	1.3	72	22	6	28

Even though Sufentanil could be given relatively much faster than Fentanyl there was the same incidence of rigidity. The induction time was faster than Fentanyl and comparable to that of Alfentanil. Cardiovascular parameters were stable.

2.

	% Patients SBP ↑ 20% OR greater			
	Intubation	Incision	Sternotomy	S.Spread
Fentanyl	0	0	32	52
Sufentanil	0	0	11	22

The haemodynamic stress response using Sufentanil was reduced 2-3 fold compared to the standard Fentanyl technique.

3.

	% Patients Requiring Phentolamine, N_2O and Nitroprusside for Control of SBP			
	Phentolamine		N_2O	Nitroprusside
	Pre CPB	CPB	Post CPB	After CPB
Fentanyl	42	47	53	21
Sufentanil	6	11	11	6

The use of supplements with Sufentanil was comparable to the high dosage Fentanyl technique.

4.

RECOVERY TIMES

	Conscious (hrs)	Ready For Extubat. (hrs)	Not Ready For Extubat. 8 Hours After Op.(%)
Fentanyl	2.1	4.6	21
Sufentanil	1.8	4.8	17

Discussion

Throughout the initial study period cardiac output and heart rate were remarkably stable. Certainly it appeared that by giving the morning pre-operative oral dose of β-blocker to those patients already taking the drug the cardiovascular system was more stable pre bypass. This effect was noticed in both groups.

Recovery of consciousness and extubatable time were similar to the standard Fentanyl method. However we felt that Sufentanil appeared to give crisper end points. The elimination half-lives of Sufentanil and Alfentanil are stated to be shorter than that of Fentanyl (Bovill and Sebel, personal communication).

It was note worthy that with Sufentanil, as with the high dose Fentanyl method, well over 90% of the total dose of the respective drug was given by bypass time. Some workers are in fact giving the total estimated anaesthetic dose of Sufentanil together with a full paralysing dose of Pancuronium as one bolus for induction. This would appear to make titration difficult with no induction dose as a yardstick of narcotic requirement.

Sufentanil versus standard Fentanyl technique

1. Sufentanil affords a faster induction time than Fentanyl with the same incidence of muscle rigidity.
2. The recovery time is similar to Fentanyl.
3. Less supplements are needed with Sufentanil to control the haemodynamic stress response.
4. Sufentanil is easier to use and appears to afford a better "narcotic anaesthesia" than Fentanyl in patients undergoing coronary artery bypass grafting operation.

Alfentanil: Comparison of a bolus technique and a constant infusion technique.

Alfentanil has a fast onset of action and a very short elimination half-life. In addition our initial study suggested a constant infusion technique for stability and ease of management. With this in mind we compared our bolus technique with an Alfentanil constant infusion technique.

Method constant infusion.

15 Patients for coronary artery operations were studied. The procedure was exactly the same as with the bolus Alfentanil technique until immediately after intubation when a constant infusion of 50 mg per hour of Alfentanil was commenced. This maximum rate was maintained pre-incision and at times of maximal surgical stress. The infusion rate was guided by the cardiovascular parameters and adjusted as one would the dial of an anaesthetic vapouriser. Vasodilators were used if indicated as described before.

Results

1.   ALFENTANIL

Percentage rise in SBP > 20%

	Intub.	Incis.	Stern.	S.Spread
BOLUS	0	0	60%	73%
INFUSION	7	7	13%	0

2.   ALFENTANIL   SUPPLEMENTATION

	Before CPB	CPB	After CPB	
	Phentolamine		N_2O	SNP
BOLUS	0	27%	47%	33%
INFUSION	0	20%	0	0

3.   ALFENTANIL   RECOVERY

Conscious hrs. postop.

BOLUS	1.4 hrs.
INFUSION	3.1 hrs.

Discussion

Remarkable cardiovascular stability was afforded using the infusion techniques. Only 7% of the patients showed rises of systolic blood pressure to 20% of control values during initial anaesthetic and surgical stresses. No rise was recorded at maximal sternal spread in contrast to the 73% incidence with the bolus technique. Use of supplements was restricted to bypass time especially in the rewarming phase and here the use of vasodilator was similar to the bolus group.

Although the rate of infusion could be reduced and sometimes stopped it was found that Alfentanil had to be given right to the end of the operation. Nevertheless the total dosage was similar in both groups. We had extrapolated the initial infusion rate from the dose required pre bypass using the bolus method as a guide.

Return of consciousness was twice as long as with the bolus method, however, all patients were extubatable within the 8 hour postoperative study period. This method gave us the greatest cardiovascular stability of the techniques so far examined.

Conclusion

1. High dose narcotic techniques afford "stress free" anaesthesia with stable cardiovascular dynamics.
2. Sufentanil appears better than Fentanyl as a complete narcotic "anaesthetic" for coronary artery bypass grafting operation.
   Possibly because the more potent the narcotic, the greater the specificity it has for the receptor site.
3. Alfentanil infusion affords, in our opinion, the most stable stress free narcotic technique so far tested. Possibly because there is a persistantly high concentration of the narcotic at the target organ.
4. More potent narcotics with shorter duration of action might possibly provide the ideal "stress free" narcotic anaesthetic agent.

References

1. Stanley, T.H., Philbin, D.M., Coggins, C.H. (1979). Fentanyl-oxygen anaesthesia for coronary artery surgery. Cardiovascular and antidiuretic hormone responses.
   Can. Anaesth. Soc. J., 26, 168.

2. Lunn, J.K., Stanley, T.H., Eisele, J., et al. (1979). High dose fentanyl anaesthesia for coronary artery surgery: Plasma fentanyl concentrations and influence on cardiovascular responses.
   Anaesth. Analg., 58, 390.

3. Hall, G.M. (1980). Fentanyl and the metabolic response to surgery.
   Br. J. Anaesth., 52, 561.

4. Hall, G.M., Young, C., et al. (1978). Substrate Mobilisation during surgery. A comparison between halothane and fentanyl anaesthesia.
   Anaesthesia, 33, 924.

5. Stanley, T.H., Berman, L., Green, O., et al. (1980). Plasma catecholamine and cortisol responses to Fentanyl-Oxygen anaesthesia for coronary artery operations.
   Anaesthesiology, 53, 87.

6. Hill, A.B., Nahrwold, M.L., et al. (1980). Prevention of rigidity during Fentanyl-oxygen induction.
   Anaesthesiology, 53, 568.

7. Comstock, M.L., Scamman, F.L., et al. (1979). Rigidity and hypercarbia on Fentanyl-oxygen induction.
   Anaesthesiology, 51, 528.

8. Waller, J., Hug, C., Nagle, D.M. (1981). Fentanyl/Oxygen anaesthesia and coronary bypass surgery.
   Anaesthesiology (In Press).

9. de Lange, S., Stanley, T.H., Boscoe, M. (1980). Comparison of Sufentanil-oxygen and Fentanyl-oxygen anaesthesia for coronary artery surgery.
   Anaesthesiology, 53, 864.

10. Stanley, T.H., Leysen, J., Niemegeers, C.J.E. (1980). The influence of Diazepam and Droperidol on C.N.S. receptor binding.
    Anaesthesiology, 53, 533.

11. De Castro, J., Van de Water, A., et al. (1979). Comparative study of cardiovascular neurological and metabolic side effects of eight narcotics in dogs.
    Acta Anaesthesiol. Belg. 30, 5.

ELECTROENCEPHALOGRAPHIC RESPONSES DURING HIGH-DOSE OPIOID ANAESTHESIA

JG BOVILL MD., FFARCS(I)., PS SEBEL MB., PhD., FFARCS(I)., A WAUQUIER PhD[*],
P ROG.

Dept. of Anaesthesia, Academic Hospital, University of Amsterdam

[*]Dept. of Pharmacology, Janssen Pharmaceutica, Beerse, Belgium.

INTRODUCTION

The use of high doses of opioids as complete anaesthetic agents in cardiac surgery has become increasingly popular during the past decade. The introduction of this technique originated in the observation by Lowenstein and his co-workers in the Massachussetts General Hospital, Boston that, in patients undergoing treatment of respiratory failure with mechanical ventilation, doses of morphine sufficient to suppress respiration had no discernable haemodynamic effects despite the large doses frequently required. They extended this observation to the use of morphine 0.5-3 mg/kg as the sole, or major component of anaesthesia for patients undergoing aortic valve replacement (1). However, although morphine in these doses gave good cardiovascular stability it was not altogether problem free. A major disadvantage, which became apparent when the technique was used for patients undergoing coronary artery surgery was a high incidence of awareness and inadequate anaesthesia. In an editorial on the subject in 1971 Lowenstein stated that "Morphine produces profound analgesia without consistently causing loss of consciousness" (2). Indeed, in the relatively fit patient who has not suffered from a chronic, low cardiac output syndrome, it may be necessary to use very high doses of morphine to abolish awareness. Doses up to 11 mg/kg have been reported (3). Such large doses result in very prolonged respiratory depression in the post-operative period.

Because of these difficulties, fentanyl was investigated as an alternative to morphine and was found to give as good or better cardiovascular stability in patients having mitral valve (4) or coronary artery surgery (5). The use of fentanyl in doses of 50-100 μg/kg appears to be devoid of many of the problems associated with the high-dose morphine technique. In particular, patient awareness and the production of unconsciousness have not been problems. To date there are only two reports in the literature of awareness occuring

during fentanyl anaesthesia (6,7). In one case (6) this occured with the
second, but not the first, of two fentanyl anaesthetics which were six days
apart. The total doses of fentanyl were similar in each case (76 and 76 µg/kg).
However diazepam was given during the first anaesthesia. The second report
(7) concerned a 41 years old woman undergoing elective mitral valve replacement,
given a total dose of fentanyl 90 µg/kg, who was aware of sounds and conver-
sation associated with sternotomy.

Despite the, by now widespread, clinical experience with high-dose fentanyl
anaesthesia in cardiac surgery there still remains a reluctance among many
anaesthetists to accept that opioids in appropriate doses can produce true
surgical anaesthesia. One method by which the question as to whether or not
opioids produce anaesthesia can be answered is to study the electroencephalographic responses during surgery with a high-dose opioid technique. The
results of such a series of investigations with fentanyl and two of its
newer analogues, sufentanil and alfentanil are presented here.

METHODS

Patients undergoing elective or emergency cardiac surgery with cardiopulmonary bypass were studied. Premedication was lorazepam 3-5 mg orally
90 min prior to surgery in all but one group of patients anaesthetized with
fentanyl 60 µg/kg, in whom morphine 10 mg intramuscularly was used. This
latter premedicant group was included to determine the influence, if any,
of lorazepam on the EEG changes occuring during fentanyl anaesthesia. After
positioning of radial artery catheter, central venous catheter and peripheral
infusions and the placement of Ag-AgCl stick on EEG electrodes, a 6 minute
control EEG recording was obtained using a Beckman Accutrace 8-channel
electroencephalograph. The amplified EEG signal from a representative sample
of patients from each anaesthetic group was also recorded on magnetic tape
for subsequent off-line computer analysis.

Following pre-oxygenation, pancuronium 2 mg was injected intravenously
(to prevent muscle rigidity) and then the appropriate dose of opioid was
administered intravenously over a 2 min period. A further 6 mg pancuronium
was given for muscle relaxation when the patient became unresponsive.
The doses of opioids used were:

Fentanyl 30-70 µg/kg

Sufentanil 15 µg/kg

Alfentanil 50-180 µg/kg followed by a continuous intravenous infusion at a rate of 500-750 µg/kg/hr.

Patients given fentanyl 30 and 50 µg/kg and 5 patients of those given fentanyl 60 ug/kg were ventilated with O_2/N_2O (F_IO_2 = 0.5), the remaining patients were ventilated with O_2/Air (F_IO_2 = 0.5). Ventilation was adjusted to maintain the PCO_2 between 35-40 mmHg.

The EEG was continuously monitored until the onset of cardiopulmonary bypass and intermittently after bypass. Because of the changes associated with bypass and hypothermia ($26^{o}C$) no analysis was made during this period. In the fentanyl group the recordings were visually analysed and classified into "EEG levels" according to a classification described by Kugler (8). These "levels" were then plotted as "narcograms" - graphical representations of the EEG. Three dimensional (0.5-15 Hz) and wideband (7 frequency bands in the range 0.5-40 Hz) power spectral analysis was performed on the signals recorded on tape using a PDP 11/E 10 computer (9).

RESULTS

The changes in the EEG during induction of anaesthesia were similar with all three opioids. The fast beta activity (13.5-25 Hz) present in the awake premedicated state disappeared and slow alpha waves (7.5-13.5 Hz) became prominent. By 30-40 sec after the start of induction these had also disappeared and were replaced by diffuse theta activity (3.5-7.5 Hz) and some delta waves (0.5-3.5 Hz), maximal in the frontal leads. By 150 sec the predominent feature was a monomorphic EEG picture of high voltage slow synchronised delta waves with almost no theta activity. This corresponds to EEG level E in the Kugler classification. Not all patients reached this level, although levels D2-3 were always seen. A representative progression of EEG changes, recorded from a patient anaesthetised with fentanyl 70 µg/kg is shown in Fig. 1. After approximately 5 minutes the EEG became more irregular, the amplitude of the delta waves decreased and theta activity again became apparent. The pattern then changed very little until the onset of cardiopulmonary bypass in patients given sufentanil 15 µg/kg or fentanyl 50-70 µg/kg. Those given fentanyl 30 µg/kg showed significantly faster activity which was often associated with classical signs of inadequate anaesthesia. The changes in EEG level in the fentanyl group are demonstrated in Fig 2, in which the mean narcograms for each dose are plotted.

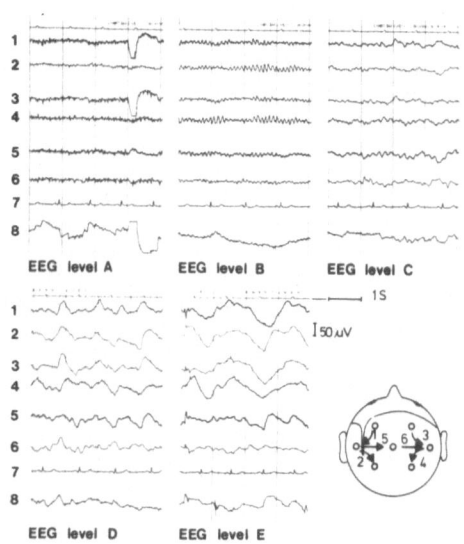

FIGURE 1. Example of EEG changes during induction of anaesthesia with
fentanyl 70 μg/kg. Premedication was lorazepam 5 mg. Lead 8 is from a
frontal derivation used specifically to detect eye movements. Lead 7
displays the ECG. EEG level A shows normal awake pattern with eyes open.
Eye movements are seen in leads 1, 3 and 8. EEG level B shows diffuse
slow alpha rhythm. Level C shows theta activity with some delta waves.
Increasing delta activity is obvious in level D, with some theta activity
still present. Level E shows synchronised high-voltage delta waves.

It can be seen that the EEG level is uninfluenced by premedication or by
the use of Nitrous oxide. The lighter "EEG response" in patients given
fentanyl 30 μg/kg is demonstrated. Patients receiving alfentanil infusion
had considerably greater variability in their EEG than these receiving
fentanyl or sufentanil. This probably reflects variation in the plasma levels
of this very short acting drug, since the infusion rate had to be frequently

114

altered to maintain a satisfactory level of surgical anaesthesia, as judged
clinically.

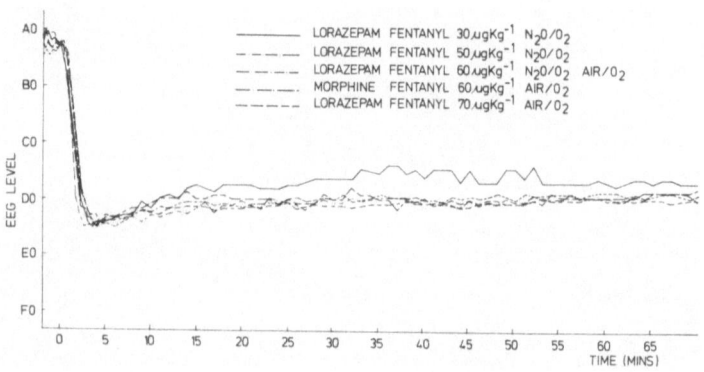

FIGURE 2. Mean narcograms for all fentanyl groups studied. The 30 μg/kg
group has a lower EEG level than the other groups from 15 minutes after
induction.

No EEG changes were observed in any patient during intubation, skin
incision or sternotomy. Following skin incision, diathermy caused considerable
interference in the EEG, although there were always sufficient uninterrupted
segments available for visual analysis. After cardiopulmonary bypass delta
activity remained evident although the amplitude was less and there was
an increase in theta activity. Occasional alpha activity was observed towards
the end of the operation in patients anaesthetised with fentanyl or sufentanil
- this disappeared when small incremental doses of opioid were given (fentanyl
250-500 μg/kg, sufentanil 100-200 μg/kg). The appearance of alpha activity
during alfentanil anaesthesia was often associated with clinical signs of
light anaesthesia and was an indication for increasing the infusion rate
and/or giving a bolus increment.

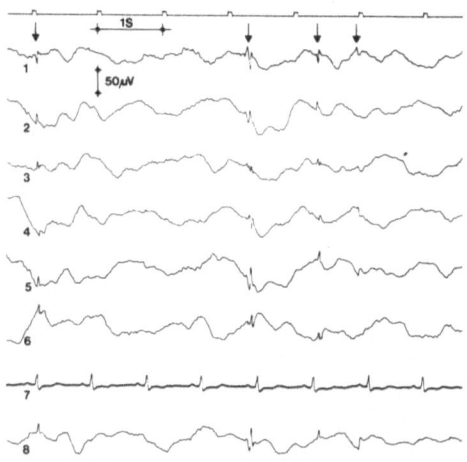

FIGURE 3. Example of sharp waves (arrowed) occuring 3 min after induction
of anaesthesia with sufentanil 15 µg/kg. The predominant EEG activity is
in the delta range. Similar sharp waves were also seen with fentanyl and
alfentanil.

Isolated sharp-wave activity was observed in all patients within 2-3
min after induction. (Fig. 3). These were mainly triphasic with an amplitude
of 10-70 µV and a period of 30-60 msec. They were most obvious in the
fronto-temporal region and occured with a frequency of 8-12 min during the
initial 10-15 min and then disappeared or were only occasionally seen.
They were never seen after cardiopulmonary bypass and were not associated
with any signs of generalised epileptic activity.

A representative example of 3-dimensional power spectral analysis, from
a patient given sufentanil 15 µg/kg is shown in Fig. 4. In the pre-induction
period there is some low-powered delta together with occasional alpha and
beta activity. The enormous increase of power in the delta band and virtual
disappearance of power in the other bands is impressively displayed. After
chest incision diathermy interference prevented continuous computer analysis.
No changes in the spectral analysis were observed following intubation or
sternotomy. The changes in the power in the various bands during alfentanil

anaesthesia are demonstrated in a different manner in Fig. 5 - this is an
example of wideband power spectral analysis.

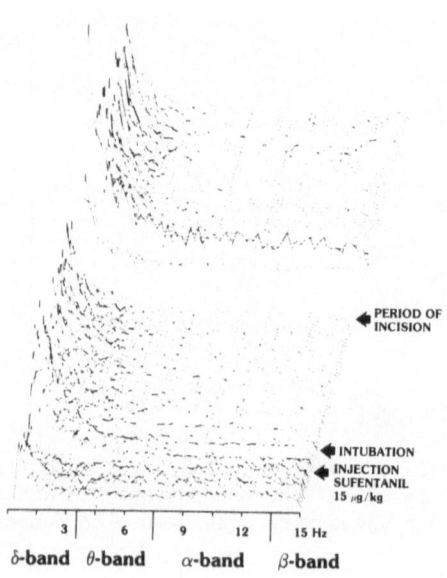

FIGURE 4. Example of a 3-dimensional power spectral analysis of the EEG
during sufentanil anaesthesia using the T_3-C_0 derivation. Power (mW) is
plotted vertically. Each line represents 1 min in time. The blank period
after incision is the result of diathermy interference. The plot demonstrates
the shift from alpha/beta activity in the awake state to high-powered delta
activity after induction.

Again the virtual disappearance of alpha and beta power can be seen accompanied
by the striking increase in delta power. The delta power was generally more
variable during alfentanil infusion than in patients given fentanyl or
sufentanil, for reasons mentioned previously. More theta activity was observed
with alfentanil than with the other drugs. The maximum delta power immediately
after induction of anaesthesia was correlated with the induction dose of
alfentanil ($r = 0.77$).

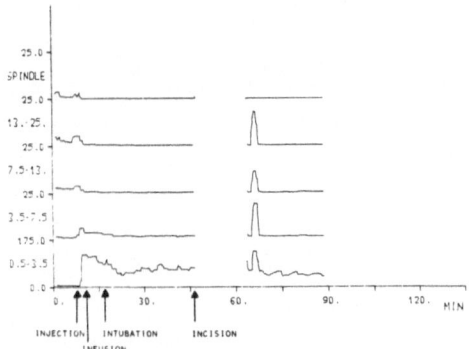

FIGURE 5. Example of wideband power spectral analysis during alfentanil anaesthesia (induction with 127 µg/kg followed by a continuous infusion at 500-750 µg/kg/hr). Time is shown on the horizontal axis. The vertical axis represents power (mW) in each frequency band: delta 0.5-3.5 Hz: theta 3.5-7.5 Hz: alpha 7.5-13 Hz: beta 13-25 Hz. The blank section after incision is caused by diathermy interference. The peaks at 65 min are also due to signal artefacts.

An advantage of wide band spectral analysis over the more spectacular 3-dimensional plots is that it allows statistical analysis to the applied, so that the change in mean power with time within a group can be calculated. Although the mean delta power decreased after induction with fentanyl and sufentanil, the contribution of delta power to total power in the EEG in the frequency range 0.5-40 Hz remained remarkably constant, especially in those patients given sufentanil (Fig. 6). Sufentanil is approximately 10 times as potent as fentanyl - 15 µg/kg is therefore equivalent to 150 µg/kg fentanyl.

118

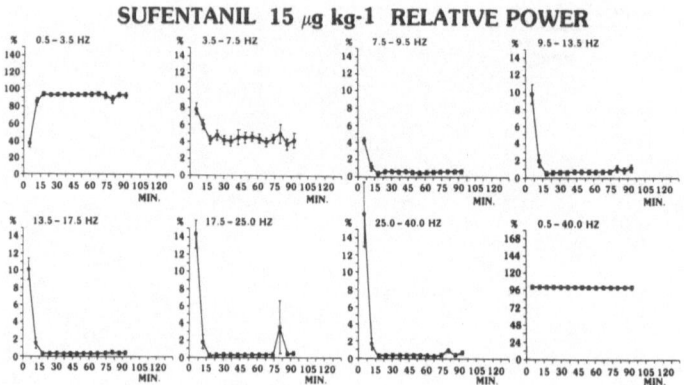

SUFENTANIL 15 µg kg-1 RELATIVE POWER

FIGURE 6. Mean (± SEM) relative contribution of the power in the various frequency bands to the total power, equalized at 100% at each time period. These results are from a group of 12 patients given sufentanil 15 µg/kg.

DISCUSSION

The EEG has been in the past only sporadically used by anaesthetists as an useful tool for investigating the effect of anaesthetic drugs. Part of the reason for this must lie in the difficulty of interpreting the raw signal. Each drug produces a different series of changes in the EEG and there is no standard feature which might be useful as a monitor of anaesthetic depth with doses in clinical usage. However, if one examines the literature on this subject carefully a general trend can be distinguished, namely a reduction in the frequency content of the EEG during surgical anaesthesia. Some drugs, e.g. cyclopropane, produce a characteristic high voltage delta wave (0.5-3.5 Hz) pattern with concentrations sufficient to produce anaesthesia. With others such a picture can only be observed at concentrations beyond these normally used clinically. Halothane 2-3% produces a dominant frequency of 10-12 Hz and irregular waves of 3-5 Hz (theta waves) only become evident with hyper-ventilation or by the addition of nitrous oxide (10).

The effects of the opioids on the EEG is characterised by high voltage delta wave activity, which is not affected by the addition of nitrous oxide

or by lorazepam premedication. The reappearance of higher frequency activity
as was observed in patients given fentanyl 30 µg/kg was often associated
with clinical signs of inadequate anaesthesia. We feel that the presence
of a predominent high amplitude delta activity in the EEG is an indication
of deep surgical anaesthesia and consider the appearance of higher frequencies
an indication of lightening anaesthesia and a signal that additional opioid
may be required.

There is a similarity between the EEG effects of these drugs and those
seen during non-REM sleep, which is also characterised by slow delta waves.
During arousal from sleep the EEG changes from a predominantly high voltage
low frequency pattern to one with low voltage high frequencies. Similar
"arousal reactions" have been reported in patients anaesthetised with
halothane in response to intubations, skin and peritoneal incision (10,11).
It seems that such changes are an indication of inadequate depth of
anaesthesia. Such changes were not observed in our patients with the exception
of some patient given the lowest dose of fentanyl.

The neurophysiological significance of the sharp waves is uncertain. They
were not associated with signs of generalised epileptic activity such as
myoclonus although this may have been masked by the use of pancuronium.
Similar sharp waves have been described in dogs following the administration
of opioids (12) and also after the injection of beta-endorphin into the
cerebral ventricles of rats (13). It is possible to demonstrate either
activation of epileptic foci or spike waves activity with all commonly used
anaesthetic agents with the exception of halothane (14).

The constancy of the delta band contribution to total EEG power and the
apparent correlation between the induction dose of alfentanil and the power
in this band suggests that this may be an useful index of anaesthetic depth
during opioid anaesthesia. Modern computer technology is rapidly producing
more sophisticated, smaller and cheaper microprocessors. It is possible
that in the not to distant future such devices may be used to provide on-line
EEG analysis and to give the anaesthetist a reliable and immediate monitor
of anaesthetic depth in the operating theatre.

REFERENCES

1. Lowenstein E, Hallowell P, Levine FH, et al. 1969. Cardiovascular responses to large doses of intravenous morphine in man. New Eng J Med 282:1389-1393.
2. Lowenstein E. 1971. Morphine anesthesia - a perspective. Anesthesiology 35:563-565.
3. Stanley TH, Gray NH, Stanford W, et al. 1973. The effects of high-dose morphine on fluid and blood requirements in open-heart operations. Anesthesiology 38:536-541.
4. Stanley TH, Webster LR. 1978. Anesthetic requirements and cardiovascular effects of fentanyl - oxygen and fentanyl - diazepam - oxygen anesthesia in man. Anesth Analg (Cleve) 57:411-416.
5. Lunn JK, Stanley TH, Eisele J, et al. 1979. High dose fentanyl anesthesia for coronary artery surgery: Plasma fentanyl concentrations and influence of nitrous oxide on cardiovascular responses. Anesth Analg (Cleve) 58: 390-395.
6. Mummaneni N, Rao TLK, Montoya A. 1980. Awareness and recall with high-dose fentanyl-oxygen anesthesia. Anesth Analg (Cleve) 59:948-949.
7. Hilgenberg JC. 1981. Intraoperative awareness during high-dose fentanyl - oxygen anesthesia. Anesthesiology 54:341-343.
8. Kugler J. 1966. Electroencephalographie in Klinik und Praxis. II. Thieme. Stuttgart. pp 53-66.
9. Wauquier A, Verheyen JL, van der Broek WAE, et al. 1979. Visual and computer-based analysis of 24 hour sleep-waking patterns in the dog. Electroenceph Clin Neurophysiol 46:33-48.
10. Backman LE, Löfström B, Widen L. 1964. Electroencephalography in halothane anaesthesia. Acta Anaesth Scan 8:115-130.
11. Oshima E, Shingu K, Mori K. 1981. EEG activity during halothane anaesthesia in man. Brit J Anaesth 53:65-72.
12. Wauquier A, van der Broeck WAE, Niemegeers CJE, et al. 1981. Effects of morphine, fentanyl, sufentanil and the short-acting morphine-like analgesic alfentanil on the EEG in dogs. Drug Development Research (in press).
13. Havlicek V, La Bella FS, Pinsky C, et al. 1980. Beta-endorphin induces general anaesthesia by an interaction with opiate receptors. Canad Anaesth Soc J 27:535-539.
14. Stockard JJ, Bickford RD. 1975. A basis and practice of neuroanaesthesia. Ed. Gordon E. Excerpta Medica. Amsterdam. pp 3-46.

The author gratefully acknowledges the permission to reproduce figures 1 and 2 from Anesthesiology and figures 3, 4 and 6 from the British Journal of Anaesthesiology.

ELECTRICAL ANESTHESIA

A. LIMOGE, Y. LOUVILLE, L. BARRITAULT, J.B. CAZALAA, A. ATINAULT

INTRODUCTION

Since 1973 we have been able to perform deep investigation in our research on the application of transcranial currents on man and we have thus developed a method of electropharmaceutical anesthesia.

During these years of experimental studies and clinical human trials, not only have we been able to find efficacious currents provoking neither initial shock, pain or unpleasant sensation, nor burns or other cutaneous damage, or muscular contractures, respiratory depression or cerebral lesion, but we have been able to locate ideal site for the electrodes and to select the most efficient drug associations at a minimum dose.

MATERIAL AND METHOD

A.   NATURE OF CURRENT

The output current is biphasic. It is composed of modulated high-frequency pulse trains (peak-to-peak intensity 250 mA, average intensity 0). The on-time of the wave trains is 3 or 4 mS, followed by a 10, 8 or 7 mS off-time. These wave trains are composed of successive impulsional waves of a particular shape: one positive impulse of high intensity and short duration, followed by a negative impulse of weak intensity and long duration adjusted in such a way that the positive surface be equal to the negative surface. The use of such a negative phase makes it possible to eliminate all risks of burns (fig. 1, 2). [19, 21]

This research was supported by U.S. Army Medical Research and Development Command Contract n° 17-75-C-5039, and INSERM Contract n° 80.3002.

122

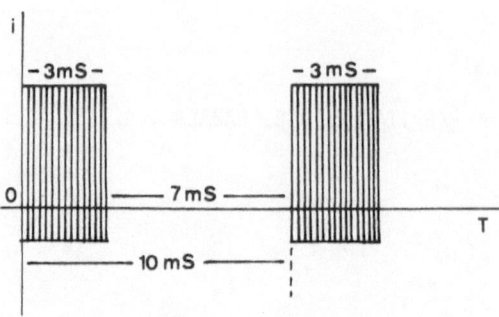

FIGURE 1

*Electric L.F. parameters are preselected (A, B
and C positions on the generator). Above drawing
shows C position : cyclic ratio 3/10 mS (A and
B positions being respectively 3/13 and 4/12 mS).*

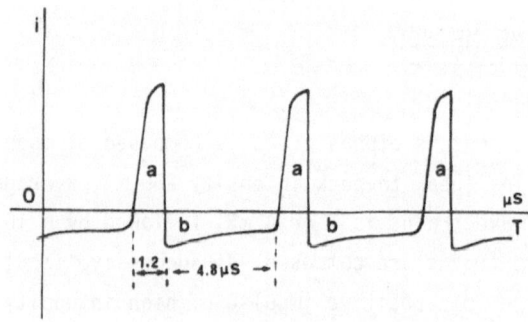

FIGURE 2

*H.F. parameters are preselected F1 and F2. This
drawing shows F1 position : $I^+ = 1.2$ µS, $I^- = 4.8$ µS
(F2 position being : $I^+ = µ2$ S, $I^- = 4$ µS).*

This type of current found its shape very progressively as the human clinical essays proceeded. The shape and cyclic ratio of the H.F. waves are of utmost importance to provoke analgesia. Various shapes of waves have been tested (triangular, rectangular, exponential), and the best result was given by the signal with an exponential ascent and acute fall. As regards the cyclic ratio of the H.F. waves, 1/5 was the best one, i.e. t'_1 = 1.2µS, and T' = 6µS (fig. 3).

B.   ELECTRODES

There are three electrodes: the frontal one is placed between the eyebrows and the two posterior ones are placed behind the mastoïd process on each side of the occiput. The intracerebral electric field thus obtained spreads on each side of the median line, but a great part of the electric current spreads over the scalp thus provoking peripheral electrostimulation (fig. 4). The use of biphasic current permits to employ "Patch ECG" self-sticking electrodes made of silver (active diameter 30 mm) (fig. 5).

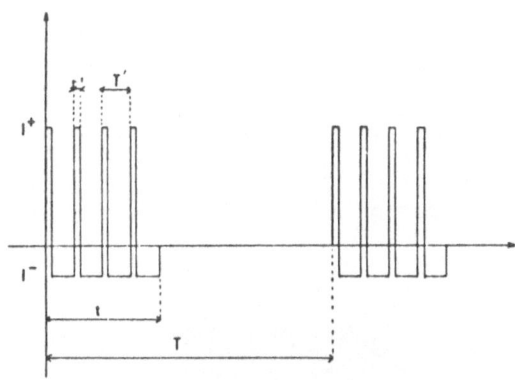

FIGURE 3

t'_1 : *high frequency on-time*

T' : *high frequency pulse duration*

t : *low frequency on-time*

T : *low frequency period*

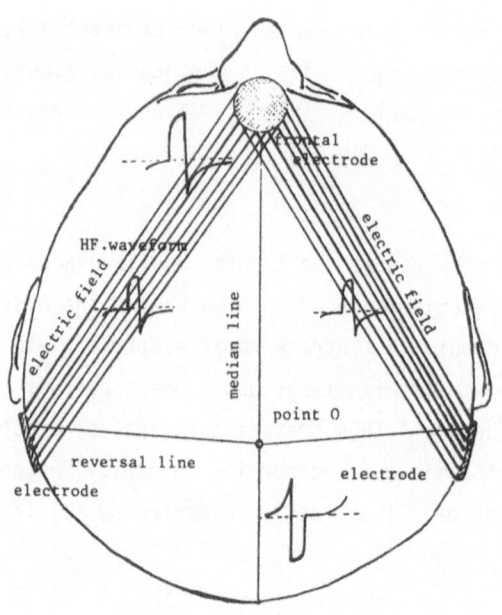

FIGURE 4

Shape of wave on the scalp

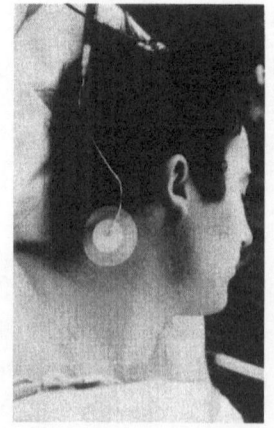

FIGURE 5

Self-sticking electrode

C.   GENERATOR

The generator for electroanesthesia has been simplified in order
to facilitate its use (fig. 6).

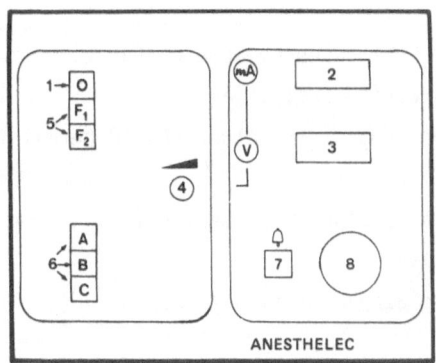

FIGURE 6

a)   *A luminous push button (1) is used to switch on or off.*

b)   *Two peak-to-peak detectors measure the amplitudes of current and
      voltage applied to the patient. These two numbers can be read*
permanently on the front face of the apparatus (2) and (3). These visual
checks permit to make sure that the contacts between skin and electrodes
are correct, and permit constant evaluation of the level of current injected.*

c)   *The potentiometer (4) permits to check the quantity of current
      injected.*

d)   *Five luminous push buttons (5) and (6) allow selection of six
      different combinations. The duty cycle of the H.F. pulse train is
adjustable by two-position switches (5). F1 position gives 1/4 H.F. cyclic
ratio, and F2 gives 1/3 H.F. cyclic ratio. The modulating pulse train is
adjustable in frequency and duty cycle (6). The modulating waveform is a
L.F. pulse train gating H.F. signal (100% modulation).*

e)   *The generator is connected to the patient by means of three cables
      (8). At the end of each is a "Patch ECG" self sticking electrode.*

D.   CHOICE OF INDUCTION DRUGS[5, 8, 22]

The drug association used for induction is composed of a neuro-leptic, a narcotic, and sometimes an analgesic, for the following reasons:

   . Security: a classic anesthetic drug must be possible at once in case of need ;

   . Each parameter must be changeable at any time (for neurovegetative protection, narcosis, analgesia) ;

   . Suppressing one drug or the other should permit to determine the real action of current.

Good results were obtained with the following combinations used during our clinical essays:

   . droperidol,   diazepam or flunitrazepam)
   . perimetazine,   "   "   "   ) *with or*
   . diethazine,   "   "   "   ) *without*
   . cyamepromazine,   "   "   "   ) *fentanyl*

It seems as though butyrophenone or phenothiazine derivates were indispensable to obtain good anesthesia.

As a conclusion to all our clinical essays, and all our biological and neurological tests, we have been in a position to establish a routine protocole for electroanesthesia and to demonstrate the advantages of this new technique.

E.   GENERAL PROTOCOLE[22]

E.1.   PREMEDICATION.

Forty five minutes before the beginning of anesthesia, intra-muscular injections of - vagolytic drug (atropine, scopolamine...),

                        - anxiolytic drug (benzodiazepine, butyrophenone...)

E.2.   SETTING OF ELECTRODES AND CURRENT.

   a) cleansing of skin
      preparation of electrodes with the gel
      location of electrodes and setting

   b) Application of current: Increase of intensity up to 300 mA (30 V. voltage). It is quite possible to apply current on patients who are fully conscious since the current we use does not provoke the slightest sensation or contracture. As the maximum effect occurs within 15 to 20 minutes, it is applied preferably before induction drugs.

E.3.   DRUG INDUCTION.

a) It is still necessary to use chemical induction on man in order to obtain optimal results from electroanesthesia. The most frequently used combination in France is the following:

. neuroleptic (droperidol 10 mg),

. hypnotic (diazepam 15 mg, or flunitrazepam 1 mg)

b) Other combinations are studied, such as Gamma OH or steroïdes (alfatesine), propanidine, ethomidate, thiopental (physiological sleep doses).

E.4.   INTUBATION.

It is performed with or without myorelaxant, but always with anesthesia of the larynx (the endotracheal probe should be covered with an anesthetic gel).

E.5.   VENTILATION.

A 50% mixture of N_2O - O_2. It has been reported that the electric current is potentialized by N_2O.

E.6.   MAINTENANCE OF ANESTHESIA.

50% mixture of N_2O -O_2 plus electric current (the parameters are changed every twenty minutes in order to avoid habituation). No further injection of induction drug should be made, except for myorelaxants. Still, in case neurovegetative protection turns out to be insufficient in spite of . the modification of the LF cyclic ratio (from A to B) ,

. the increase of intensity ,

. the modification of the HF cyclic ratio (from F1 to F2), a neuroleptic drug is injected (C.07 mg/kg of droperidol).

In case the patient recovers consciousness without any sign of pain, he is given a 5 mg injection of diazepam (hypnotic).

In case he shows signs of pain despite the neuroleptic injection, he is given a 0.1 mg injection of fentanyl (analgesic). In such case the electrical technique is a failure.

If the patient receives no more current, whatever the reason may be, the analgesic effect will decrease within a few minutes and surgery will be no longer possible, but it will be easy to carry it on with a classical technique.

E.7.   CLINICAL MONITORING. It is the same as for any general anesthesia.

RESULTS

Of course, we would not go as far as saying that miracles have been achieved. Still, over 10 000 operations have been performed with our method in France and not the slightest accident has ever been reported, although this method was applied for various types of surgery, and often on patients presenting a pathological background.

A.   PER-OPERATIVE PHASE[17, 20, 22]
. All patients have been operated on as scheduled, in satisfactory conditions, without any secondary effects such as muscle contractures of trunk, limbs or face, or abnormal bleeding.

. The use of electrocoagulation did not provoke any change in wave trains or any waking up of the patient.

. Operative spirometry on non-curarized patients was always normal : an average flow of 7 l/mn with a frequency of 15 mn (total flow 500 ml).

. No watering of the eyes was reported. Pupils were in a state of myosis. Eye movements sometimes appeared in the course of anesthesia, just like what is noted during REM sleep.

. Some signs are very typical of **electroanesthesia** : swallowing movements, chewing of the probe, slight limb movements, this without any sign of pain.

. Body temperature decreased by 1 to 2° C as compared with the initial temperature for a 3 h. anesthesia.

. Electroanesthesia provoked neither cardio-vascular arhythmia nor conduction disturbances. A slight increase in the arterial pressure was often reported (10 to 20 mmHg), and sometimes a slight increase of the pulse (5 to 10 pulses/sec.).

B.   RECOVERY OF CONSCIOUSNESS AND POST-OPERATIVE PHASE
As soon as the current is stopped, ventilation comes spontaneously back to normal in a satisfactory manner, thus allowing extubation. The patients understand and execute orders and recover full consciousness very quickly. Still, they remain in a state of indifference for a period of 6 to 12 hours after return to bed, with periods of sleep if not stimulated. Most of the patients have a good night's sleep without any hypnotic drug, which is rather exceptional.

Complaints of patients after electroanesthesia are less frequent in our recovery-room than for other patients operated on with narco-neuroleptanalgesia. The operative wound being less painful, they need no antalgic, i.e. even less drugs[14].

Body temperature comes back to normal within an hour with intense shivering on the part of the patient, and increases up to a maximum of 39° C three to seven hours after surgery.

Intestinal transit comes back to normal fairly quickly and diuresis turns out to be more satisfactory than with conventional anesthesia.

After a very septic type of operation (urology for instance), septicemia or local abcesses are less frequently reported, probably because defence mechanisms are not so much inhibited.

DISCUSSION

In spite of all the theoretical advantages of electroanesthesia, the technique is liable to be criticized and it is not easily adopted because it is not yet "pure" electroanesthesia. This method requires a number of supplements, especially induction which is performed with butyrophenone (droperidol) and benzodiazepine (diazepam) compounds, or maintenance of anesthesia which is made with a 50% mixture of nitrous oxide-oxygen.

Accordingly, the use of supplements along with electrical currents clouds the issue, and the anesthesiologists rightly want to know if the current is really necessary and what part electricity is playing in this technique.

From a scientific standpoint, all prior evaluation of electroanesthesia, as used on the human, could be considered as anecdotal and as a metaphysical curiosity based on the subjective interpretation of results by surgeon- and anesthesiologist-searchers. In order to avoid these criticisms and in order to evaluate the real action of current during the course of surgery, the analgesic effect of current was studied: the quantities of analgesic drugs used on 30 patients receiving electric current or not were compared.

The 30 patients were divided into two groups (group I submitted to electroanesthesia, group II submitted to classical anesthesia). Both groups received the same induction drugs and underwent the same type of surgery with the same anesthesiologist (table I).

POPULATION STUDIED	TYPE OF SURGERY	INDUCTION
GROUP I EA n = 15 { M = 10 F = 5 average age 51 av. weight 69 kg	prostatic adenoma ..... 5 pyelolithotomy ..... 4 anti-reflux ureterovesical implantation 2 partial cystectomy ..... 1 coraliform calculus ..... 1 silicone ureteroplasty ... 1 nephro-ureterectomy 1	drop. 20 mg diaz. 20 mg phen. 2 mg
GROUP II CA n = 15 { M = 9 F = 6 average age 53 av. weight 70.5 kg	prostatic adenoma ..... 6 pyelolithotomy ..... 3 anti-reflux ureterovesical implantation 4 nephro-ureterectomy ..... 1 epididymo-deferential anastomosis 1	drop. 20 mg diaz. 20 mg phen. 2 mg

TABLE I - GROUPS STUDIED

Studying the quantities of drugs injected during the course of surgery in the two groups (table II) shows that: GROUP I received no further injection of droperidol or diazepam and that further injections of phenoperidine were very light ($3.62 \cdot 10^{-5}$ mg/kg/mn), whereas GROUP II required further injections of droperidol ($2.17 \cdot 10^{-3}$ mg/kg/mn), of diazepam ($2.36 \cdot 10^{-4}$ mg/kg/mn), and particularly of phenoperidine ($30.73 \cdot 10^{-5}$ mg/kg/mn).

The statistical comparison of phenoperidine doses injected after induction is very significant ($p < 0.001$). Which tends to ascertain the analgesic effect of electric current.

	GROUP I (EA)	GROUP II (CA)	
Droperidol (10^{-3} mg/kg/mn)	0	2.17	
Diazepam (10^{-4} mg/kg/mn)	0	2.36	
Phenoperidine (10^{-5} mg/kg/mn)	3.62	30.73	$p < 0.001$
Pancuronium (10^{-4} mg/kg/mn)	4.83	4.16	N.S.

TABLE II - QUANTITIES OF DRUGS INJECTED DURING SURGERY

This analgesic effect is lasting. Post-operative antalgy is reported to last up to sixteen hours (av.).

As mentioned above, complaints in the recovery-room are less frequent after electroanesthesia. Two groups of 100 patients each were compared (one group EA, one group CA):

. Identical drug induction in both groups (droperidol 20 mg, diazepam 20 mg, phenoperidine 2 mg).

. Maintenance in group I (CA) with medicamentous injections, and with electric current in group II (EA).

. The study was made during the first sixteen hours after surgery (table III).

. The patient was to receive 15 mg of pentazocin in case of complaint.

. Group I (CA) received an average of 29.7 mg of pentazocin per head, whereas group II (EA) received 8.1 mg per head (average), i.e. 3.6 times less. The analysis of detailed results in table III show that in group I (CA) only 20% patients did not require any analgesic injection whereas they were 65% in group II (EA).

. The difference between the two groups is statistically significant ($p < 0.001$).

This remaining and prolonged antalgy is perhaps the most important advantage of the method.

PENTAZOCIN INJECTIONS	GROUP I (CA) n = 100	GROUP II (EA) n = 100
none	20	65
One (15 mg)	14	20
Two (30 mg)	28	11
Three (45 mg)	24	4
Four (60 mg)	14	0
Average per head (mg)	29.7 ($\pm$19.88)	8.1 ($\pm$12.69)

Table III - Comparison of two groups receiving pentazocin during the first 16 hours after surgery

CONCLUSION

Anesthesiology tries to establish a fair balance between the different drugs used in order to provide the patient with sufficient anesthesia and less intoxication. Still, the duration of surgery is more and more important (micro-surgery, cardiac surgery, peripheral neuro-surgery, etc.) and requires more and more important doses of drugs. The balance between physical and chemical methods, permitting a decrease in the use of drugs and an equally good quality of anesthesia and protection of the patient is therefore a rather attractive prospect.

To sum it up one can say that electroanesthesia is now part of the various possibilities at the disposal of anesthesiologists. It is especially recommended in major surgery of long duration (over three hours), and with patients suffering from renal, hepatic or respiratory insufficiency, or in a state of shock or myasthenia, or suffering from septicemia or acute infection. It is not to be recommended for short duration surgery or on patients suffering from serious arterial hypertension with decrease of vascular elasticity.

The method is still to be perfected because the mode of action of the current is not yet perfectly elucidated. We hope to grasp the full understanding of its mechanism by studying biological and neurological tests and by performing double-blind studies.

REFERENCES

1. LIMOGE A. Etude expérimentale de l'électroanesthésie générale. Thèse, Paris 1970, 189 pages.
2. LIMOGE A. Obstetric electroanalgesia. The nervous system and electric currents, vol. 2. NL. WULFSOHN and A. Sances Jr. Ed., 189-193, 1971.
3. M. CARA, M. CARA-BEURTON, C. DEBRAS, A. LIMOGE. Essai d'anesthésie électrique chez l'homme. Ann. Anesth. Franç. XIII, 4, 1972.
4. M. CARA, C. DEBRAS, B. DUFOUR, A. LIMOGE. Long-term electromedical anesthesia in forty cases of major urological surgery. In Electro-therapeutic Sleep and Electroanesthesia. Vol. III, F.M. Wageneder and R. H. Germann Ed., Graz, 1974, pp. 221-230.
5. COEYTAUX R. A propos de 145 anesthésies électromédicales en chirurgie urologique. Thèse de Médecine, Faculté de Médecine de Necker-Enfants-Malades, 1974.

6. DEBRAS C., COEYTAUX R., LIMOGE A., CARA M. Electromedicamentous anesthesia in men. Preliminary results. Rev. I.E.S.A., n° 18-19 July 1974, p. 57-68.

7. LIMOGE A. An introduction to electroanesthesia. Univ. Park Press, Baltimore(Md), 1975.

8. DEBRAS C., LIMOGE A., VIGREUX G., LEPRESLE E., DUFOUR B., BONNAUD P., CARA M. Comparison between drug associations used in electropharmaceutical anesthesia. In Electrotherapeutic Sleep and Electroanesthesia, Masson Publ. , Paris-New-York, 1978, pp. 103-108.

9. MIGNE J., MARCHER K, LE GUILLOU A., LEPRESLE E., COEYTAUX R., DEBRAS C. Dosage of glucose, LDH, catecholamines, lactate and pyruvate during and after electropharmaceutical anesthesia. Op. cit. n° 26, pp. 156-160.

10. DEBRAS C., MARCHER K., COEYTAUX R., VIGREUX G., CARA M. Dosage of the main cellular enzymes during electropharmaceutical anesthesia. Op. cit. pp. 149-155.

11. MIGNE J., ATINAULT A. , VIGREUX G., LE GUILLOU A., DEBRAS C., CARA M. Dosage of histamine, serotonine and bradykinine during and after electropharmaceutical anesthesia. Op. cit. pp. 161-165.

12. MANNE J. Physiological examinations before and after electroanesthesia. Op. cit. pp. 175-179.

13. LOUVILLE Y., FLORENT C., FIEMEYER A., JARREAU M., CARA M. Electropharmaceutical anesthesia in thoracic surgery. Op. cit. pp. 134-140.

14. VIGREUX G., LEPRESLE E., ATINAULT A. , CUKIER J., BEURTON D., SIMON N., CARA M. Interest of electropharmaceutical anesthesia for post-operative consequences. Op. cit. pp. 128-133.

15. LOUVILLE Y., FLORENT C., CARA M. Hemodynamic measurements during electropharmaceutical anesthesia. Op. cit. pp. 166-174.

16. COEYTAUX R., LE GUILLOU A., DEBRAS C., CLAUDE J.M., VACANT J. Evaluation of efficacity of electropharmaceutical anesthesia. Op. cit. pp. 121-127.

17. BARALE F., KUNEGEL P., GILLET M., MILLERET P. Results of our experimentation about electroanesthesia in digestive surgery. Op. cit. pp. 141-148.

18. LIMOGE A., DEBRAS C., COEYTAUX R., CARA M. Electrical technique for
     electroanesthesia concerning 300 operations. Op. cit. pp. 109-120.
19. LIMOGE A., BOISGONTIER M.T. Characteristics of electric currents used
     in human anesthesiology. NATO ASI Series, Advanced Technology,
     Sijthoff and Noordhoff Publ., the Netherlands, 1979, pp. 443-452.
20. COEYTAUX R., ATINAULT A., CAZALAA J.B., LOUVILLE Y. Etude à double-
     insu de l'efficacité de l'anesthésie électromédicamenteuse. In
     Agressologie, 1977, 18, 4, pp. 213-219.
21. ATINAULT A., CAZALAA J.B., COEYTAUX R., LOUVILLE Y. Comparaison à
     double-insu de deux modalités d'application du courant de Limoge
     en anesthésie électrique. In Agressologie, 1978, 19, 6, pp. 393-397.
22. DEBRAS C., ARTIGUES J.M., GILLET G. et al. Use of Limoge's current
     in human anesthesiology. Op. cit. 19, pp. 447-465.

x x x
x   x
x

PROTECTION OF THE ISCHEMIC BRAIN

B.F. Cohn

As a direct result of the high levels attained in cardiopulmonary intensive care during the 1950's and 60's, attention has been focused upon brain resuscitation and protection. Today even with the best of care more than 10-20 % of the survivors of cardiac arrest or head injury sustain some degree of permanent brain damage (1, 2-5, 7).
This fact has given impetus to a deeper study of the problem whereby new insights into the mechanisms behind ischemic-anoxic insults as well as new concepts in therapy have evolved. It is the autor's intention to briefly sketch some of these changes and to present the concept of "brain protective agents" based upon a discussion of barbiturates and of etomidate.

PHYSIOLOGICAL MECHANISMS OF THE BRAIN

In order to fully comprehend the events occurring during an ischemic-anoxic insult as well as the aim of the therapeutic measures taken, it is necessary to briefly review some of the essential dynamic mechanisms at play within the cranium.

The human brain, of all body organs, is particularly sensative to ischemic-anoxic insults for three fundamental reasons. First, it has a high resting level of energy utilization. Secondly, the brain has no oxygen stores and only low energy reserves and, finally, in contrast to other tissues, the capillaries in the brain, even at rest, are all open so that further recruitment is not possible (8, 9).
The crux of the matter rests upon the supply of oxygen and glucose to the brain.
This in turn is dependant upon the cerebral blood flow, both global and regional, the hemoglobin content and quality, and the oxygen saturation of the blood.

These are all in relation to each other as shown by the formula

Oxygen Availability = CBF x So_2/100 x   Hb   x 1.39

whereby, So_2 = oxygen saturation of hemoglobin

Hb = hemoglobin concentration

1.39 = amount of oxygen in mls. carried by 1 gm. of hemoglobin

Cerebral blood flow is only indirectly affected by cardiovascular function as it is protected from fluctuations in systemic arterial and venous pressure by the mechanism known as cerebral autoregulation. The extracranial vascular system expresses its influence upon cerebral blood flow through the mean arterial and jugular venous pressures according to their relationship to cerebral perfusion pressure as shown by the formula: CPP = mean arterial pressure minus intracranial pressure or jugular venous pressure-depending upon which of the latter two has the highest value.

Cerebral autoregulation in turn is responsive to differences in cerebral perfusion pressure. It maintains a constant cerebral blood flow despite fluctuations within more or less constant upper and lower threshold limits in the normotensive person. These limits are probably equally raised in the hypertensive individual. Above and below these threshold levels CBF varies passively, if not linearly, with perfusion pressure (9, 10).

Autoregulation is also greatly influenced by blood arterial carbon dioxide levels. Hypercarbia leads to vasodilation and hypocarbia results in vasoconstriction. Additionally it is responsive to brain tissue pH, but not to hydrogen ion fluctuation in the blood because the blood brain barrier, if intact, is relatively impermeable to charged ions resulting from metabolic alkalosis or acidosis. The brain only becomes affected by these changes after a long delay (1, 10). In contrast, cerebral vasculature is much less responsive to changes in arterial oxygen content. Levels must be reduced to around 50 torr before significant vasodilation occurs.

In summation, a few critical pressures. When cerebral perfusion pressure falls below 60 torr, all other things being normal, CBF begins to decline. If it surpasses a critical threshold level of 30-40 torr, CBF will be significantly decreased and may abruptly cease (2, 7, 9, 11). Intracranial pressure is generally considered to be normal up until 15

torr and does not significantly reduce overall CBF until it reaches
30-40 torr; again all other factors being normal (11). Jugular venous
pressure is of no significance provided it remains below intracranial
pressure. The human brain is more resistant to pure hypoxemia than
orginally thought as seen by the fact that cerebral vasculature only
dilates, as stated before, around 50 torr and arterial levels of 30 torr
can be tolerated provided cerebral perfusion is maintained. Evidently
the brain tissue is normally supplied with an excess of oxygen (9, 11).
Finally, the CPP limits which will exceed autoregulatory control in
the normotensive are respectively 130 torr for the upper and 60 torr for
the lower threshold values. Naturally all of the above values pertain to
essentially normal conditions and are greatly altered by pathological
states.

THE CLASSIFICATION OF BRAIN HYPOXIA

Although there are numerous ways in which to classify ischemia-
hypoxia, the following classification lends itself best to an understanding
of the terminology used when referring to the dynamics involved in brain
protection and resuscitation.

Ischemic hypoxia: is merely a reduction or cessation of blood flow to
the tissues, as exemplified by cardiac arrest of hemorrhagic shock.

Hypoxic hypoxia: implies an insufficeincy in oxygen supply to an adequate
circulation resulting in a reduction in oxygen saturation of the
hemoglobin and decreased oxygen plasma tension, as occurs with suffocation.

Anemic hypoxia: is a disturbance in hemoglobin function or a reduction
in hemoglobin content, examples being carbon monoxide intoxication and
anemia.

Histotoxic hypoxia: is the bluckage of oxidative systems by noxic or
toxic agents such as occurs with cyanide poisoning.

The definition of hypoxia itself, according tn Siesjo (12) io simply
"a reduction in available oxygen to levels that are insufficient to
maintain function, metabolism, or structure" and anoxia is "the complete
absence of oxygen".

The treatment of the various types of cerebral hypoxia is basically
straight forward. Oxygen is supplied in hypoxic hypoxia, blood or packed
cell for anemic hypoxia, and antidotes for histotoxic hypoxia.

Ischemic hypoxia is another story and it is this which is the central problem in this discussion.

Ischemia is definable in similar terms to that of hypoxia. It is (13) a "reduction of CBF to levels insufficient to sustain normal cerebral function, metabolism or structure. It can be global affecting the whole brain, as with cardiac arrest or hypotension, or focal, with an interruption of flow only to certain regions, as occurs with stroke. In addition each of these can be complete, meaning a total stop in circulation, exemplified by cardiac arrest, or incomplete meaning a reduction but not cessation of flow, as occurs with hypotension. Head trauma takes an unusual position within these definitions because depending upon circumstances it can be any of these combinations (14, 15).

When looking at the biochemical changes occuring in brain cells during ischemic anoxia it is important to keep in mind several unique features of brain metabolism (16, 17, 18).

1. The brain has high energy requirements. Consequently, energy stores as well as oxygen are rapidly depleted.

2. Under normal circumstances glucose and oxygen are the only substrates. Only under special circumstances are other exogenous substrates used.

3. About 90 % of the glucose is oxidized to carbon dioxide and water, the rest becoming pyruvate. Only 5-8 % of the pyruvate is converted to lactate.

4. Metabolic energy is conserved in the form of ATP which is used for the work tasks of the cells, mainly active transport, biosynthesis, and ion transport.

5. The brain is markedly non-homogenous with respect to anatomy, circulation and metabolism.

6. Neurotransmitters, by acting through synaptic transmission have potent effects upon brain metabolism, circulation and membrane function. Most likely they account for the coupling of normal brain circulation and metabolism.

7. Biogenic amines are involved in synaptic transmission and may modulate neuronal receptivity to stimuli.

8. Brain electrical and functional neurological dysfunction can and does occur without evidence of brain metabolic failure during and after ischemic-anoxic insults. This is due to failure of neurotransmitter function and not energy metabolism failure.

9. The fact that therapy administered after the insult can ameliorate the neurological deficits sustained signifies that a substantial portion of the damage occurs after the restitution of circulation. This fact alone has completely altered the therapeutic approach to circulatory arrest and other forms of ischemic-anoxic insults.

THE BIOCHEMICS OF ISCHEMIA-ANOXIA

What happens during and ischemic-anoxic insult? Cardiac arrest will be used as an example because this gives the most clear-cut picture (7, 13, 16, 17, 19, 20).
Globally, the events occuring must be separated into two phases; the initial ischemic phase and the following reperfusion phase arising after cardiac resuscitation. The reasons for this delineation will become evident in the following discussion.

The ischemic-anoxic phase

During this period there is an abrupt arrest of circulation and a rapid depletion of oxygen. Consciousness is lost within 10 seconds time. Glucose and glycogen stores are rapidly exhausted and even low energy anaerobic metabolism, due to the lack of ATP and phosphocreatine, ceases within 4-5 minutes. As all energy requiring reactions come to a halt sodium/potassium pumps in the cell membranes fail and intracellular osmolality increases paving the way for possible intracellular edema formation. These are the general changes occuring.

In the meantime various metabolic dysregulations arise. First, there is an energy metabolism failure. While the normal oxidative processes are arrested anaerobic glycolysis increases seven-fold. Consequently, lactacidosis and a subsequent fall in pH is seen. This reaction continues for as long as glucose, glycogen, ATP and phosphocreatine reocrves are present. Among other things, acidosis promotes edema formation and mitochondrial damage.

Lipid metabolism is also disturbed. During the ischemia free fatty acids accumulate. The greatest increase is seen in arachidonic and stearic acids. The FFA's are very damaging substances as will be evidenced in the reperfusion phase.

A third biochemical dysruption occurs in the form of a neurotransmitter failure and involves the tricarboxylic acid cycle and catacholamines. The TCA cycle dysfunction leads to a decrease in nearly all its intermediates and linked excitatory amino acids while there is simultaneously an increase in the neuron-depressive amino acids such as gamma-amino-butyric acid and alanine. The catecholamines, specifically dompamine, noradrenaline, and serotinin, all decrease because, among other things, they require oxygen for their synthesis.

Another potentially dangerous change also occurs during the ischemic phase. The basis is laid for free radical formation activity (13, 19, 20, 21, 22, 23). Free radicals are atoms or molecules with a single, unpaired electron in their outer shell, They are extemely reactive and aggressive compounds and particularly attack unsaturated fatty acids in the phospholipids of membranes - especially those of the mitochondria and endoplasmic reticulum. Normally they are rapidly quenched by inhibitors called either bioantioxidants or free radical scavengers as soon as they are produced by so-called activators. Under anaerobic conditions this balance is disturbed and the bioantioxidants decrease while, due to the lack of oxygen, there is a total reduction of the elements of the electron transport chain. This creates a sort of free radical emergency state giving rise to initiators of free radical peroxidation reactions. With reperfusion, the oxygen molecules present react with the reduced electron transport chain at other sites than the normal cytochrome C oxidase steps. Via the formation of H_2O_2 free radicals are generated and in the absence of sufficient scavengers do their damage.

A final occurance during the ischemic phase is that there is a shift in brain water from the extra- into the intracellular compartment. This is generally due to the increase in osmolality, Na/K pump failure and alterations in membrane permeability which, in addition to other things, is reflected in the increase of free fatty acids.

Naturally, if circulation is not restored the processes initiated during this ischemic phase lead to cellular death.

As mentioned earlier the free fatty acids are particularly damaging. FFA's inhibit mitochondrial oxidation, uncouple oxidative phosphorylation, and cause a decrease in membrane glucose transport. Furthermore the arachidonic acid which increases to a great extent is a precurser in prostaglandin synthesis and this latter substance may be involved in

creating vasospasm. Finally the FFA's also increase blood coagulability
and affect synaptic transmission in a negative fashion. They may reflect
phosphilipid breakdown in the subcellular membranes which means that
these membranes become prone to peroxidative attack. Since oxygen supply
is restored, though as is evident by the above in insufficient amounts
in some areas, the highly active free radicals are formed. Due to the
lack of bioantioxidants the balance is disturbed and these atoms and
molecules further the damage which is already in progress.

Thus in the reflow stage, what one sees is a multifocal hypoperfusion-
hypoxia combined with a hypermetabolic state.

If resuscitation is successful, the so-called reflow phase is begun.
This is characterized by the restoration of circulation and the resupplying
of the two essential substrates oxygen and glucose (glycogen). There
appears to be a generalized hyperemia, but actually this is a false
impression. Although the total flow to brain increases there is
precapillary A-V shunting, and the no-reflow phenomenon limits regional
circulation. This latter state results from vasospasm, increased local
tissue pressure, capillary compression and intra-vascular coagulation.
This is all made worse by the fact that certain areas also lose their
reactivity to carbon dioxide changes and autoregulation is disturbed.
The end result is a non-homogenous flow throughout the brain with areas
of hyper- and of hypo-perfusion.

Simultaneously, while the above cerebral blood flow disturbances are
occuring, there is an increase in catecholamines. By themselves or
indirectly by their stimulation of the production of cyclic AMP, a
hypermetabolic state is created. These two cause a three fold increase
in oxygen utilization, an increase in glycolysis with further production
of lacatcidosis, an increased proteolysis and decreased protein synthesis,
and further an increase in free fatty acids due to increased lipolysis.

Basically the brain damage sustained by ischemic-hypoxic insults
depends upon a multiplicity of factors. In essence though, four factors
are essential. To begin with not only is the degree of hypoxia, but also
the presence or absence of hypotension important. As stated earlier,
humans are fairly resistant to pure hypoxia. When accompanied by
hypotension, even moderate degrees of hypoxia can be damaging. The
reason for this is that in incomplete ischemic-hypoxia basic substrates

such as glucose and oxygen are delivered to the brain tissues, but in insufficient amounts. Consequently, both damaging processes requiring substrate, such as glycolysis, as well as other processes needing oxygen molecules, such as free radical membrane peroxidation, continue working for longer periods than in complete circulatory arrest. In the latter instance these processes would be self-limiting. Consequently, neuronal damage resulting from stroke can sometimes be more extensive than that occuring after cardiac arrest (6, 16, 24, 25).

Another factor of importance is the duration of ischemia-hypoxia. The decisive factor for whether a MAP of 30-40 torr will result in cerebral ischemia and/or irreversible shock is the duration of time during which it is sustained. Normally, complete neurological clinical recovery is likely if a cardiac arrest does not exceed a duration of 5-7 minutes at normal body temperature (16, 26).

A third essential factor is the restoration of adequate, more or less homogenous flow throughout the brain. Unfortunately, after a number of acute conditions, such as head trauma, stroke, and episodes of hypoxia and/or hypotension, there is regional loss of autoregulation and carbon dioxide reactivity combined with a reduction in brain tissue oxygen tension. These non-homogenous low-flow states are equivalent to a multiple micro-stroke syndrome (7, 17, 27).

Finally, the timing of instituation of therapy is essential to recovery. It is evident that if therapy is initiated either before and/or during the insult - as with the cerebral protection methods - of within one hour postischemia - which is the basis of cerebral resuscitation - a substantial degree of amelioration of neurological deficit can be achieved (28, 29, 30, 31, 32).

CEREBRAL RESUSCITATION - PROTECTION

What does cerebral resuscitation or protection entail? In essence, it consists, first and foremost, in treating the underlying etiological factors, such as cardiac arrest, and in getting the body back into homeostasis by means of adequate generalized intensive care therapy. This entails such things as maintenance of MAP at 90-110 torr, avoiding episodes of hyper- and hypotension, keeping $PaCO_2$ around 100 torr, $PaCO_2$

between 25-35 torr, proper fluid and electrolyte balance, and all the rest. In addition, more specific brain therapies may be applied. These are:

a. steroids: to stabilize membranes, reduce edema, scavenge free radicals, decrease CSF production, and increase seizure threshold (1).

b. reflow promotion: by arterial hypertension for 6 hours, brief carotid perfusions, normovolemic hemodiution with dextran 40, and anticoagulation with heparine. All these methods have variable results and can be harmful.

c. osmotherapy: basically to dehydrate normal and ischemic brain tissue and so limit edema formation. Glycerol and mannitol reduce ICP and seem to independantly increase CBF in regional ischemic zones. Also used are hypertonic solutions, dextrans, albumins, and sometimes supplimentation with diuretics.

d. temperature regulation: hypothermia is effective if induced before an insult or during it. It reduces metabolism, inflammatory response to injury, decreases edema formation, protects enzyme activity, retards ATP depletion and prevents lactacidemia development. Hyperthermia is harmful to the brain. Hypothermia is justified if given with barbiturates which reduce shivering and are additive.

e. surgery: carotid enarterectomy, microvascular by-pass procedures, decompressive operations for raised ICP, etc.

f. neuron protective agents

As can be seen specific brain protective drugs are only one facet of a whole arsenal of neuron-saving measures.

There have been a number of agents which have at one time or another been accredited with having neuroprotective properties. Mainly these substances only work by one mechanism alone and their true neuron-saving qualities are still in doubt. Furthermore they only appear to function under given specific circumstances. Even immobilization with pavulon, as seen in monkey experiments, has been shown th have an ameliorating effect upon neurological deficits if combined with ventialtion (33, 1).

How do these so-called neuron protecting agents work? Since barbiturates have been accredited by one investigator or another with all of the possible mechanisms of action, it will be used as the example (1, 9, 34, 35).

First, barbiturates are supposed to improve the distribution of CBF by exercising a vasoconstrictive action upon cerebral vessels in the non-ischemic regions. This results in the so-called reverse steal phenomenon whereby blood is shunted into low perfusion areas. This is primarily supposed to be functional in focal ischemia. Furthermore by lowering raised ICP it also promotes global cerebral perfusion.

Second, barbiturates if given in high enough doses can reduce cerebral oxygen utilization by 50 %. Thus during hypoxic periods, it spares oxygen for vital cellular processes. It is believed that the decreased utilization of oxygen probably reflects decreased neuronal function rather tahn actual cell metabolism reduction. One theory is that this effect is achieved by barbiturate action upon catacholamines and cyclic AMP.

The improved redistribution of flow plus the reduction in oxygen utilization consequently serves to bring supply and demand more into balance. This is especially important in the reperfusion phase with its low flow and hypermetabolism.

Third, barbiturates appear to have free radical scavenging properties. Actually this has only been verified for thiopental, is perhaps also true of methohexital, but has as yet to be demonstrated for pentobarbitol and phenobarbital.

Fourth, barbiturates are believed to stabilize membranes. Perhaps by being lipid-soluble they incorporate themselves into the membrane itself, though no one knows how this is done. Evidence of this is seen by the fact that barbiturates prevent both the extracellular rise in K^+ normally taking place during ischemia (41, 42) as well as the calcium influx across synaptosomal membranes, which if occuring, would stimulate presynaptic neurotransmitter release (42). They also stabilize lysosomal enzymes preventing the release of acid hydrolases which destroy cellular components (41).

Fifth, barbiturates also reduce intra- and extra-cellular edema formation (17, 19). This occurs in conjunction with the above mechanisms.

Sixth, barbiturates both prevent and suppress convulsive hyperactivity with its subsequent lactacidosis. They can be administered to burst suppression levels, or even isoelectric levels if necessary.

Nevertheless, it must be emphasized that all of these supposed mechanisms giving rise to the protective action of barbiturates are controversal and that the real true reason for their neuron-saving effect has still to be established.

Turning to animal experimentation, what appears to be substantiated with respect to the brain preotective properties of barbiturates? (14, 18, 34, 36, 37, 38, 39). To begin with, barbiturates clearly do ameliorate neuronal damage due to focal ischemia. The reduction in infarction appears to be dose related. In addition, they also reduce the formation of cerebral edema. Their action with respect to protection from global ischemia is less clear due to conflicting reports, criticism of the animal models and methods used, and the difficulty in separating out the effect due to other life-support measures needed to sustain the animals. Still, there does appear to be a tendency towards protection sufficient enough for some investigators, the Pittsburgh group in particular, to feel justified in setting up clinical barbiturate trials in humans. What evidence there is seems to clearly establish that protection is both dose and time related thereby necessitating large barbiturate dosages and the institution of therapy either before, during, or within one hours time postischemia.

In contrast, humans evidence for barbiturate protection is sparse and often based upon supposition. That barbiturates can play a valuable role in the reduction of elevated intracranial pressure - which is indirectly a brain protective effect-has been clearly established by, among others, the clinical work of Shapiro, Marshall, Rockoff and Smith (44, 45, 46). This now is an accepted therapeutic measure in many neurosurgical units. There is a lack of information as to barbiturate value in ameliorating focal ischemia, although its preventive application before surgical procedures seems to imply, though not statistically, a beneficial effect (43, 47, 48). Large randomized controlled studies in this area are necessary (49). There are only a few studies of barbiturate use in the resuscitative treatment of cerebral ischemia (32, 50, 51).The Pittsburgh initiated multi-institutional non-randomized, uncontrolled feasibility trial which investigated 40 patients is the largest and best documented of this group (32). By administering a large bolus injection of either thiopental of thioamylal these investigators found that in 22 patients with cardiac arrest times varying from 5-22 minutes duration 64 % recovered completely without neurological sequelae. The anticipated response under identical therapeutic circumstances without the use of barbiturates would have been 10 % or less. Nevertheless, in this as well as in other clinical trials, it is difficult to separate out what is due to generalized cerebral supportive care measures and what can be attributed to barbiturates. Further, randomized, controlled, large scale clinical investigations are still necessary.

One thing clearly established by the clinical studies using barbiturates for cerebral protection is that its administration is fraught with difficulties. A particular problem is the dosage required and the means of administration. Whether it is given protectively or resuscitatively, that is, before, during or after the insult, depends upon the indications and circumstances at the time. Some give barbiturates as a single loading dose (Pittsburgh- 32), others as a loading dose followed by a continuous maintenance infusion (Stanford, Heidelburg- 50, 51), while there are those who administer barbiturates first as intermittent infusions to a given loading level and then continue with intermittent infusions according to response (San Diego- 44, 45, 46). The dosages or barbiturates used to load the patients vary considerably extending from the high 30-50 mg/kg used by the Pittsburgh multi-institutional study through the 12-15 mg/kg used in Stanford and Heidelberg to the 3-5 mg/kg found necessary to reduce intracranial pressures in San Diego (45, 46). Infusion rates and plasma concentration parameters also vary as no one seems to know the minimum plasma concentration necessary for barbiturate brain protection. Dosage and administration is generally directed by preventing unnecessary accumulation by intermittent sampling of plasma for barbiturates and by using other parameters reflecting effect, such as, burst suppression or iso-electric EEG levels, reduction of intracranial pressure, and/or immobilization of the patient.

Long duration infusions of high doses of barbiturates necessary for cerebral protection have also shown that high dosage have different pharmacokinetics than low dosages. For example, in low dosages there is first-order elimination of the drugs whereby the rate of elimination and elimination half-life are linear - that is, constant regardless of plasma concentration. With high dosages and long infusions, there is a change over to non-linear elimination whereby the rate of elimination varies with the plasma concentration. The end result is a decrease in the rate of elimination and an increase of elimination half-life with the subsequent danger of attaining high plasma barbiturates levels (52).

Another problem is acute tolerance, a situation whereby repeated administrations of a drug leads to functional and metabolic tolerance to succeeding doses. Consequently, increasingly larger dosages are necessary to achieve the same effect. Barbiturates demonstrate this characteristic (53). The mechanism behind this effect is unknown but there are indications that it may lie at the calcium influx level where barbiturates are known to be active (42).

A further problem is that barbiturates produce active metabolites which in long term administration may add to their effect. Pentobarbital, for example, is one of the metabolites arising with the long duration administration of thiopental (52).

Clinical and animal experience has also brought to light complicating side effects arising due to the use of high protective doses of barbiturates. Often due to the cardiovascular depressent effect of these dosages supportive dopamine infusions or vasopressors, like nor-epinephrine, are necessary. Hypothermia is also a problem. Temperatures generally drop only to around $33^{o}C$ levels, but sometimes warrent warming-up measures in order to stop further decline. Several instances of barbiturate hepatitis have been encountered. In a series of 8 patients treated with thiopental infusions for 6-15 days duration by Wiedermann et al (51) three developed icterus attributed to this barbiturate. The same group of patients also developed erythemas and anaphylactic reactions are not unknown with barbiturates. A Stanford investigation had serious bradycardie problems needing pacemaker support and two instances of unexplainable adult respiratory destress syndromes (50). Thus it is evident that the administration of barbiturates in dosages required for cerebral protection brings with it serious complications (44, 45, 46, 51, 32).

Primarily because of the dangers inherent in high doses of barbiturates there has been a search for other potentially brain protective agents with similar properties but less complications or side-effects. Etomidate, a highly potent short-acting hypnotic, is beginning to show signs of falling into this category. The safety of this drug has been already well established in clinical practice. It is believed to have a therapeutic index which is 5-10 times greater than other known hypnotics (54, 55). In addition it has minimal cardiovascular or respiratory depressive effects (56, 57), releases no histamine (58, 59), is not tetrogenically active (60), and has as yet to demonstrate either organ toxicity or harmful side-effects. Furthermore etomidate can be administered either in bolus form or by continuous infusion and does not appear to show cummulation nor produce active metabolites (60, 54).

Apart from all these advantages, etomidate also exercises several effects upon the brain which are similar to those of barbiturates. To begin with it changes the EEG in nearly an identical sequence and pattern (61, 62). Neuronal functional activity can be reduced to burst suppression levels either by it alone or in conjunction with moderate hypothermia (63). Laboratory and clinical investigations have also established it's anticonvulsive properties. In animal experiments (64, 65) etomidate has proved effective against both electrically and chemically produced tonic and clonic seizures. This action exceeds the period of hypnosis since the animals were stimulated 30-60 minutes after the administration of etomidate at a time when they had already recovered from its effects. Further substantiation is seen by a clinical trial performed by Van der Starre (64) upon 12 patients in status epilepticus. Five of the cases were due to underlying neurological disorders while seven appeared after craniotomy. Success was booked in all cases.
He gave an initial dose of 0.2 mg/kg i.v., followed, as required in 10 patients, by half doses up to a maximum of three times at intervals of 10-15 minutes in response to the return of seizure activity. Thus, with both postoperative as well as with therapy resistant status epilepticus patients, etomidate appears to be capable of effectively controlling seizure activity and of preventing seizure return. Further investigation is naturally necessary. The anticonvulsive action of etomidate is suspected of being related to its GABA-mimetic properties (64, 65).

Another similarity of etomidate to that of barbiturates is its effect upon cerebral oxygen utilization, blood flow and intracranial pressure. Etomidate will reduce cerebral oxygen consumption to approximately the same degree as thiopental - namely by 46 % in clinical tests when both were administered (66). In addition it is also capable of lowering cerebral blood flow, though to a lesser extent, to approximately 34 % as compared to 45 % with thiopentone (66). Naturally, as is to be expected, etomidate also lowers intracranial pressure. In an experiment upon patients with increased intracranial pressures, Schulte (67)

compared the effects of a single bolus of 0.3 mg/kg of etomidate to that
of 6 mg/kg of thiopentone. Both drugs decreased the ICP by 27 %. The big
difference was that the thiopentone caused a greater and more prolonged
drop in arterial blood pressure with the result that the cerebral perfusion
pressure also declined. Due to its cardiovascular stability the drop in
blood pressure with etomodate at this dosage was minimal so that cerebral
perfusion pressure was relatively unaffected. In both instances ICP
returned to the initial values after 20 minutes time. Although not of
consequence for these patients studied by Schulte, there can be instances
of severly limited cerebral perfusion when such differences in CPP can
be important.

Direct evidence pointing to the neuron-saving potential of etomidate
is infortunately scarce. Only a few animal experiments, all of them on
small rodent models and done in the laboratory of Janssen Pharmaceutica
can be offered as evidence of this property (68). Nevertheless, these
experiments seem to imply that etomidate is effective against complete
global ischemia, hypoxic hypoxia, histotoxic anoxia and (personal
communication) ischemic hypoxia. Also in all of these investigations
etomidate was compared to thiopental and methohexital. Of the three
etomidate was the only drug consistently effective at sub-hypnotic
doses. As yet there is no solid explanation for this potential brain
protective action of etomidate, but preliminary work (69) seems to
imply that it may in some unknown way be tied in with the suppression
of arachidonic acid during and after ischemia. In any case, if this
neuron-saving property turns out to be true, and taking into account
that the drug, like barbiturates, also provides immobilization, reduction
of the cerebral metabolic rate of oxygen consumption, and decreases
intracranial pressure and CBF while maintaining CPP due to its
cardiovascular stability - one can only conclude that it most certainly
warrents extensive study. Although at the present time more experimental
animal investigation is necessary, due to its proven benign attributes
at supposedly effective dosages, clinical investigation is also justified.

In conclusion it must be said that although there is extensive
material available concerning the brain protective potential of
barbiturates, nothing, aside from its beneficial effect upon raised
intracranial pressure, is definitely proven. Part of the difficulty lies
in the drug's severe clinical side effects, such as cardiovascular

collapse, which greatly limit its use. In addition, the establishment of both good clinical and experimental ischemic-hypoxic models is still a problem. The interaction with other brain supportive measures during preventive and resuscitative therapy makes the evaluation of barbiturates all the more difficult. No doubt a drug like etomidate will have similar problems when tested in the clinical situation, although its lack of complicating side effects is a decided advantage. Let us hope that in the near future these problems will be overcome and that good randomized controlled clinical trials and further biochemical advances will be forthcoming. Then and only then will we be able to decide for once and for all whether the existence of true brain protective agents is fact or fiction!

LITERATURE LIST

1. Safar, P., Bleyaert, A., Nemoto, E.M., et al: Resuscitation after global brain ischemia-anoxia. Critical Care Medicine, 6 (no. 4): 215, 1978.

2. Bares, D., Caronna, T.J., Cartlidge, N.E.F., et al: A prospective study of nontraumatic coma: methods and results in 310 patients. Ann. Neurol. 2: 211, 1977.

3. Bell, J.A., Hodgson, J.H.F.: Coma after cardiac arrest. Brain, 97: 361, 1974.

4. Bengtsson, M., et al: A psychiatric-psychological investigation of patients who had survived circulatory arrest. Acta Psychiat Scand, 45: 327, 1969.

5. Willoughby, J.O., Leach, B.G.: Relation of neurological findings after cardiac arrest to outcome. Br. Med. J., 19: 437, 1974.

6. Safar, P.: Introduction: on the evolution of brain resuscitation. Crit. Care Med., 6 (no. 4): 199, 1978.

7. Safar, P.: Pathophysiology and Resuscitation after Global Brain Ischemia. International Anesthesiology Clinics (Management of Acute Intracranial Disasters), 17 (no. 2 & 3): 240, 1979.

8. Siesjo, B.K., et al: Hypoxia and cerebral metabolism: in a basis and practice of Neuroanaesthesia. Exerpta Medica. (Ed. Emeric Gordon) p. 47, 1975.

9. Ping, F.C., Jenkins, L.C.: Protection of the brain from hypoxia:
   A Review. Canad. Anaesth. Soc. J., 25 (no. 6): 468, 1978.

10. Campkin, T.V., Turner, J.M.: The cerebral circulation (Chapt. 1):
    in Neurosurgical Anaesthesia and Intensive Care. Butterworths,
    London-Boston. P. 3-16, 1980.

11. Campkin, T.V., Turner, J.M.: Reduction of Intracranial Pressure
    (Chapt. 7); in Neurosurgical Anaesthesia and Intensive Care.
    Butterworths, London-Boston. p. 103,1980.

12. Siesjö, B.K.: Ischemia (Chapt. 14); in Brain Energy Metabolism.
    John Wiley & Sons, New York. p. 398, 1978.

13. Siesjö, B.K.: Ischemia (Chapt. 15); in Brain energy Metabolism
    John Wiley and Sons, New York. p. 453, 1978.

14. Enevoldsen, E.M., et al: Dynamic changes in regional CBF, intra-
    ventricular pressure, CSF pH and lactic levels during the acute
    phase of head injury. J. Neurosurg. 44: 191, 1976.

15. Fieschi, C., et al: Regional cerebral blood flow and intraventric-
    ular pressure in acute head injuries. J. Neurol. Neurosurg. Psych.
    37: 1378, 1974.

16. Nilsson, B., Norberg, K., Siesjö, B.K.: Biochemical events in
    cerebral ischaemia. Br. j. Anaesth. 47: 751, 1975.

17. Nemoto, E.M.: Pathogenesis of cerebral ischemia-anoxia. Crit. Care
    Med., 6 (no. 4): 203, 1978.

18. Smith, A.L.: Barbiturate protection in cerebral hypoxia.
    Anesthesiology, 47: 285, 1977.

19. O'Brien, M.D.: Ischemic Cerebral Edema. A Review: Stroke, 10 (no. 6):
    623, 1979.

20. Majewska, M.D., Str0nsznajder, J., Lazarewicz, J.: Effect of
    ischemic anoxia and barbiturate anesthesia on free radical oxidation
    of mitochondrial phospholipids. Brain Research, 158: 423, 1978.

21. Demopoulos, H.B.: Control of free radicals in biologic systems.
    Fed. Proc., 32: 1903, 1973.

22. Butterfield, J., Jr., McGraw, P.: Free radical pathology. Stroke,
    9 (no. 5): 443, 1978.

23. Flamm, E.S., et al: Free radicals in cerebral ischemia. Stroke, 9 (no. 5): 443, 1978.

24. Kovach, A.G.B., Sandor, P.: Cerebral blood flow and brain function during hypotension and shock. Annu. Rev. Physiol., 38: 571, 1976.

25. Siesjö, B.K., et al: Brain metabolism in the ctitically ill. Crit. Care Med. 4: 283, 1976.

26. Brierly, J.B.: The neuropathology of brain hypoxia; in Scientific Foundations of Neurology (eds. Critchley, M., O'Leary, J.L., & Jennett, B.). Heinemann, London. p. 243, 1972.

27. Ames, A., III, Wright, R.L., et al: Cerebral ischemia. II. The no-reflow phenomenon. Am. J. Pathol. 52: 437, 1968.

28. Miller, J.R., Myers, R.E.: Neurological effects of systemic circulatory arrest in the monkey. Neurology, 20: 715, 1970.

29. Nemoto, E.M., Bleyaert, A.L., et al: Global brain ischemia: a reproducible monkey model. Stroke 8: 558, 1977.

30. Hossman, V., Hossmann, K.A.: REturn of neuronal functions after prolonged cardiac arrest. Brain Res., 60: 423, 1973.

31. Hossmann, K.A., Zimmermann, V.: Resuscitation of the monkey brain after 1 h complete ischemia. I. Physiological and morphological observations. Brain Res. 81: 59, 1974.

32. Brevik, H., Safar, P., et al: Clinical feasibility trials of barbiturate therapy after cardiac arrest. Crit. Care Med., 6 (no. 4): 228, 1978.

33. Bleyaert, A.L., Safar, P., et al: Amelioration of postischemic brain damage in the monkey by immobilization and controlled ventilation. Crit. Care Med. 6: 112, 1978.

34. Belopavlovic, M., Buchthal, A.: Barbiturate therapy in cerebral ischaemia. Anesthesia, 35: 235, 1980.

35. Steen, P.A., Michenfelder, J.D.: Mechanisms of barbiturate protection. Anesthesiology, 53 (no. 3): 183, 1980.

36. Michenfelder, J.D., Milde, J.H.: Cerebral protection by anesthetics during ischemia (a review). Resuscitation, 4: 219, 1975.

37. Smith, A.L., Marque, J.: Anesthetics and cerebral edema. Anesthesiology, 45: 64, 1976.

38. Lawner, P., Laurent, J., et al: Attenuation of ischemic brain edema by pentobarbital after carotid ligation in the gerbil. Stroke 10 (no. 6): 644, 1979.

39. Simeone, F.A., et al: Ischemic brain edema: Comparative effects of barbiturates and hypothermia. Stroke, 10 (no. 1): 8, 1979.

40. Astrup, J. Nordström, L.H., Rehncrona, S.: Rate of rise in extra-cellular potassium in the ischemic rat brain and the effect of preischemic metabolic rate: evidence for a specific effect of phenobarbitone. Acta Neurol. Scand. (Suppl.) 64: 148, 1977.

41. Stolke, D., Seidel, B.U., Hartmann, N.: Barbiturate treatment and membrane stability of subcellular organelles. Anaesthesist, 29: 539, 1980.

42. Leslie, S.W., et al: Acute and chronic effects of barbiturates on depolarization - induced calcium influx into rat synaptosomes. Brain Research, 185: 409, 1980.

43. Hoff, J.T., et al: Barbiturates for protection from cerebral ischemia in aneurysm surgery; in Cerebral Function, Metabolism, and Circulation. (Ed. Ingvar, D.H., Lassen, N.) Munksgaard - Copenhagen, p. 158, 1977.

44. Marshall, L.F., Smith, R.W., Shapiro, H.M.: The outcome with aggressive treatment in severe head injureis. Part 1. The significance of intracranial pressure monitoring. J. Neurosurg. 50: 20, 1979.

45. Marshall, L.F., Smith, R.W., Shapiro, H.M.: The outcome with aggressive treatment in severe head injuries. Part 2. Acute and chronic barbiturate administration in the management of head injury. J. Neurosurg. 50: 26, 1979.

46. Rockoff, M.A., Marshall, L.F., Shapiro, H.M.: High-dose barbiturate therapy in humans: A clinical review of 60 patients. Annals of Neurosurg.: 6 (no. 3): 194, 1979.

47. Belopavlovic, M., Buchthal, A.: Barbiturate therapy in the management of cerebral ischaemia. Anaesthesia, 35: 271, 1980.

154

48. Belopavlovic, M., Buchthal, A.: Cerebral function monitoring for
    assessment of barbiturate therapy under moderate hypothermia in
    cerebral aneurysm surgery. Acta Anaesthesiologica Belgia 31: 93, 1980.

49. Astrup, J.: Barbiturate protection in focal cerebral ischemia.
    Scand. J. Clin. Lab. Invest., 40: 201, 1980.

50. Rosenthal, M.H., Larson, C.P.: Protection of the brain from
    progressive ischemia. Western Journal of Medicine, 128: 145, 1978.

51. Wiedermann, K., et al: Barbiturate infusion in severe brain
    trauma: A preliminary report. Anaesthesia, Intensive therapie ein
    noodvall medicine. 4: 303, 1980.

52. Stanski, D.R., et al: Phramacokinetics of high-dose thiopental
    used in cerebral resuscitation. Anaesthesiology, 53 (no. 2): 169,
    1980.

53. Altenburg, B.M., Michenfelder, J.D., Theye, R.A.: Acute tolerance
    to thiopental in canine cerebral oxygen consumption studies.
    Anesthesiology, 31: 443, 1969.

54. Janssen, P.A.J.: De chemie van etomidaat; in Hypnomidate (etomidaat)
    een nieuw intraveneus hypnoticum, Janssen symposiumverslag,
    Utrecht, Utrecht. p. 5, 1978.

55. Reneman, R.S.: De experimentele farmacologie van etomidaat; in
    Hypnomidate (etomidaat) een nieuw intraveneus hypnoticum, Janssen
    symposiumverslag, Utrecht, p. 11, 1978.

56. Brückner, J.B., et al: Untersuchungen zur Wirkung von Etomidate auf
    den Krieslauf des Menschen. Anaesthesist, 23: 322, 1974.

57. Rifat, K. et al: Effects de l'étomidate sur la ventilation et les
    gaz du sang. Ann. Anesth. Franc. 17: 1217, 1976.

58. Doenicke, A., et al: Histamine release after intravenous application
    of short-acting hypnotics. Br. J. Anaesth. 45: 1097, 1973.

59. Doenick, A., Lorenz, W.: Etude de l'histaminémie in vivo pendant
    l'anesthésie. Ann. Anesth. Franc., 17: 219, 1976.

60. Kay, B.: A dose-response relationship for etomidate with some
    observations on cummulation. Br. J. ANaesth., 48: 213, 1976.

61. Kugler, J., Doenicke, A., Laub, M.: The EEG after etomidat; Anaesthesiology and Resuscitation. 106: 31, 1977.

62. Ghoneim, M.M., Yamada, T.: Etomidate: A clinical and electro-encephalographic comparison with thiopental. Anesthesia and Analgesia, Curr. Res., 56: 479, 1977.

63. Massant, J., et al: Hypothermia and etomidate. Electroencephalographic aspects. Proceedings, Belgian Congress of Anesthesiology. Acta anaesth. Belg. (suppl.) 31: 275, 1980.

64. Wauquier, A., Ashton, D., Van der Starre, P.: Anticonvulsant profile of etomidate, a non-barbiturate hypnotic. 11th Epilepsy International Symposium, Firenze. Abstracts p. 135, 1979.

65. Wauquier, A., Ashton, D. et al: Etomidate: a non-barbiturate hypnotic, anticonvulsant, anti-anoxic, and brain protective actions in animals. Symposium über Anäeshtesie bei cerebralen Krampfanfällen und Intensivtherapie der Status epilepticus, Bielefeld, Bundesrepublik, Deutschland, 1979.

66. Renou, A.M., Vernhiet, J., et al: Cerebral blood flow and metabolism during etomidate anaesthesia in man. Br. J. Anaesth. 50: 1047, 1978.

67. Schulte am Esch, et al: The influence of intravenous anaesthetic agents on primarily increased intracranial pressure. Acta Neuro-chirurgioa, 45: 15, 1978.

68. Wauquier, A., et al: Anti-hypoxic effects of etomidate, thiopental and methohexital. Archives internationales de Pharmacodynamie et de Therapie. 249 (no. 2): 330, 1981.

69. Nemato, E.M., et al: Efficacy of therapies and attenuation of brain free fatty acid (FFA) liberation during global ischemia. Wolf Creek II Conference, KEy West, Fla. Nov. 14.15, 1980.

PROTECTION OF THE ISCHEMIC MYOCARDIUM

W. FLAMENG

Interruption of coronary flow and subsequent myocardial ischemia are still inherent to most operative techniques in cardiac
surgery. However, several interventions leading to improved
myocardial tolerance to ischemia are developed recently.
Because all these interventions are based on metabolic and
subcellular alterations in the ischemic myocardium, knowledge
of these biochemical and ultrastructural changes are indispensable.

At first glance, the non perfused heart should be able to cover
its energy demand by anaerobically available energy pools.
Unfortunately this is not so, the anaerobic production of
ATP from glycolysis never accounts for more than 7 % of the
normal aerobic requirements for energy (1).

After coronary perfusion is stopped, myocardial oxygen reserve is used up within 8 seconds (PO_2 decreases below 5 mm Hg)
and this shuts down oxydative phosphorilation. Consequently
the pool of creatine phosphate (CP) is used for resynthesis
of ATP but this reserve will be consumed very fast.
As ATP decreases, the ATP-inhibiton of phosphofructokinase
stops and glycolytic flux increases. However, lactate accu-
mulates and produces intracellular acidosis, which together
with elevated levels of AMP, inhibits phosphofructokinase
activity. Also glyceraldehyde 3 phosphate dehydrogenase is
inhibited by lactate accumulation glycolysis decreases and
lactate levels off. So, anaerobic metabolism covers only
65 - 70 % of total anaerobic demand.

A first approach to interfere with the process of ischemia
is directed toward this energy demand-supply balance.
The components of myocardial energy demand are :
1. basic metabolism
2. metabolism for electrophysiological "ignition-processes"
   at the outer membrane.
3. metabolism at the contractile system
4. metabolism for the inactivation of the calcium ions
   in the sarcoplasmatic reticulum being essential for
   the contraction.

Normally the metabolism of the contractile system is by far
the biggest. A first possibility to protect the myocardium
during aortic cross clamping is hypothermia.
We know that myocardial metabolism decreases exponentially
with decreasing temperature. This technique is considered
as a "classical" technique of myocardial protection.
It can be performed by general cooling to 25°C with the heart
lung machine followed by topical cooling (filling the peri-
cardial cavity with a iced slush) after crossclamping the
aorta. Mean septal temperatures of 20°C are reached.
However, a strong tension of the myocardium remains during
a heart arrest induced only by low temperature (2) because
the contractile system is not at all inactivated. This costs
energy which we wand to save. Therefore cardioplegia (i.e.
heart arrest) was propagated. Many cardioplegic solutions
are regularly used today. One of the oldes is the Kirsch solution which contained only Mg, procaïne and sorbitol.
Later Bretschneider (2) developed a better solution which was
calcium free and had a low sodium content with addition of
0,2 % procaïne. In our clinic we use the St. Thomas solution,
developed by the group of Hearse in London (3).
The composition of this solution resembles very well that of
extracellular fluid but there is a high potassium content
and procaïne is also added. We compared the two methods
(topical cooling alone and St. Thomas cardioplegia) in two
groups of patients undergoing aortic valve replacement.

As indices of myocardial ischemia and injury we used :

1) ultrastructural changes in the myocardium before and after aortic crossclamping and

2) biochemical alterations in high energy phosphates and glycogen content of the tissue and

3) intra and postoperative serial serum determinations of the CK - MB - isoenzyme.

Regarding the ultrastructure of the myocardium, we know that injury due to acute ischemia is reflected by structural changes in the mitochondria (4).

These structural alterations go through different stages according to the progression of ischemia and subsequent reperfusion. Slight damage is reflected by the disappearance of the typical osmiophilic granules in the mitochondrial matrix. This occurs already after a few minutes of ischemia. More severe damage is represented by matrix clearing, breakage of the cristae and even disruption of inner and outer membranes. Finally the irreversible stage of damage occurs when large granules of precipitated calcium (Jennings granules) are found in the mitochondria.

We dertermined semiquantitatively the percentage of damaged mitochondria in transmural left ventricular biopsies taken before and after aortic crossclamping. In none of the patients we found irreversible damaged mitochondria. However, the percentage severly damaged mitochondria was 20 % in the topical cooling group and only 5 % in the cardioplegia group ($p < 0,05$). This corresponds well with the biochemical data. ATP, CP and glycogen content was measured in comparable biopsies. In both groups ATP was unaffected after ischemia ($P > 0,05$) but CP and glycogen was significantly decreased in the postischemic biopsy in the topical cooling group ($p < 0,05$). This was not the case in the cardioplegia group. The CK-MB washout was slightly but nog significantly greater ($p > 0,05$) in the group with cooling alone. Myocardial temperature was the same in both groups : 20°C.

Figure 1.

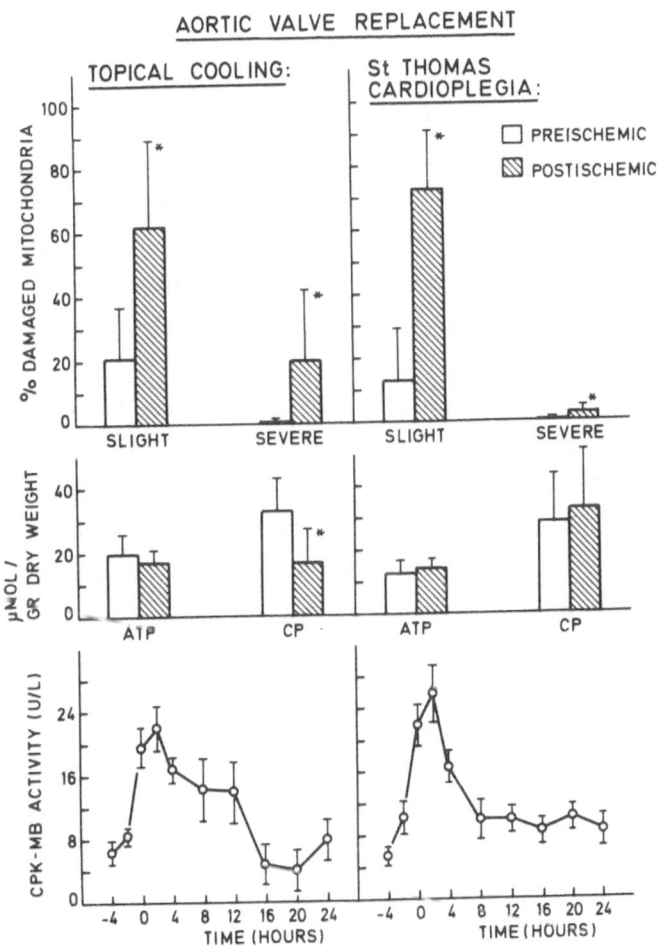

These findings demonstrate that cooling of the immediately
arrested heart provides a better protection to ischemia.
Indeed, in the arrested state, very little energy production
is needed to meet the basal requirements of keeping myocardial metabolic processes and membrane gradients intact.

These low energy needs of arrest are reduced further by hypothermia (5) :

Arrested heart	37°C	1 ml O_2/100 g./min.
Arrested heart	22°C	0,3 ml O_2/100 g./min.
Fibrillating heart	22°C	2 ml O_2/100 g./min.

When we go back to the anaerobic metabolism of the heart, we
learned that the intracellular acidosis, due to accumulation
of lactate causes much trouble to the ischemic myocardium.
Intracellular hydrogen ions displace calcium from its binding
sites on troponin and depress contractility in a few minutes.
Several enzymatic processes are inhibites by acidosis and lactate : phosphofructokinase and glyceraldehyde 3 phosphate
dehydrogenase.
Consequently glycolysis is inhibited and that means further
decrease of anaerobic ATP production. Also, an acid pH opti-
mum for lysosomal enzymes is created. Beside the nefast accumulation of lactate there is also accumulation of inorganic
phosphate (which is not incorporated in ATP) and which will
bind to calcium and precipitate. As we will discuss later,
this will decrease availability of calcium for excitation
contraction coupling which in turn may be responsible for
early pump failure.
It would be beneficial to the ischemic heart if these metabolites are washed out at regular intervals after ischemia.
The next protective technique i.e. intermittent aortic crossclamping is based on these considerations.
Several surgical interventions allow intermittent release of
aortic crossclamping. The best example thereof being aorto-
coronarty bypass grafting. To perform a distal anastomosis
(between the saphenous vein and the coronary artery) a cross
clamp time of approximately 10 minutes is required. Thereafter the myocardium can be reperfused and during that time
the proximal anastomosis (between the graft and the aorta)
can be performed using only tangential clamping of the aorta.
This may be repeated for every graft.

We studied myocardial metabolism and ultrastructure during
this type of operation in 42 patients. Again left ventricular biopsies were studied.

The biopsies were taken at the start and at the end of cardiopulmonary bypass. Additionally coronary sinus and arterial
blood was sampled during every reperfusion period and analysed for lactate, potassium, inorganic phosphate and oxygen
content. Initially, even before cardiopulmonary bypass is
started, lactate production and a loss of inorganic phosphate
is found. This indicates that the myocardium of these patients
with severe coronary heart disease is already to some extend
ischemic. After every crossclamping, there is a definite
washout of lactate, inorganic phosphate and potassium.
Potassium is lost because the sodium pump in the cell membrane
is compromised by an inhibition of the Na - K - ATP ase.
After the cardiopulmonary bypass is stopped, there is no more
lactate production nor loss of inorganic phosphate.
Ultrastructurally the percentage severely damaged mitochondria
in the postischemic biopsy is very low : 3 % in the subepi-
and 5 % in the subendocardium.
Myocardial tissue ATP is slightly but not significantly decreased in the second biopsy (p>0,05) and CP content is unchanged. This indicates preservation of high energy phosphates by this technique. Glycogen is significantly reduced
to 68 % of its initial level as can be expected. Figure 2.

These findings show that intermittent reperfusion prevent
significant damage under almost normothermic conditions :
32 - 35°C.

In contract to hypothermia, cardioplegia and intermittent
reperfusion, pretreatment with pharmacological agents is a
largely unexplored approach to protection of the ischemic
myocardium during cardiac surgery.
Several modes of pharmacological protection are indicated by
typical metabolic and structural changes that take place
during and after anoxyc cardiac arrest.

162

Figure 2.

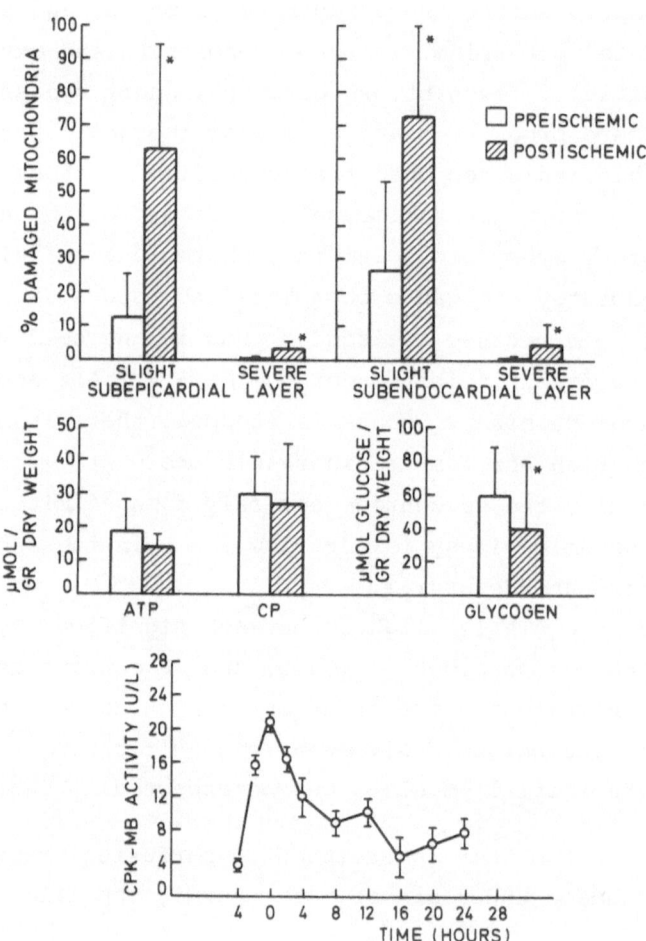

AORTOCORONARY BYPASS GRAFTING
INTERMITTENT CROSS CLAMPING (32-34°C)

As for real cardioplegia, reduction of ATP depletion during arrest may be achieved by pretreatment with metabolic inhibitors.

Beta-blocking agents (propranolol) has been shown to decrease
myocardial oxygen consumption and to block catecholamine-
induced ATP depletion in the anoxic arrested heart.
Endogenous release of catecholamines is one of the early consequences of myocardial ischemia.
Experimentally propranolol has reduced infarct size after coronary occlusion (6).
Verapamil, a powerful calcium antagonist apparently improves
recovery of function and increases ATP and CP compared with
non pretreated ischemic hearts.
This protective action seems to be due to a decrease in energy demand prior to and during ischemia rather than to a blocking of calcium influx during reperfusion (7,8).
Also Fentanyl prevents excessive breakdown of energy rich
phosphates and high anaerobic production rate of lactate by
decreasing the energy demand of the ischemic myocardium (9).

Another biochemical aspect of ischemia concerns the low levels
of adenine nucleotides in the postischemic heart : if adenine
nucleotides are lost during ischemia, how are they restored ?
The normal pathway is the novo synthesis. The limiting factor
seems to be ribose 5 phosphate.
This can arise when glucose is metabolized through the pen-
tose shunt. The activation of this pathway is probably the
main basis of long term adenine nucleotide restitution after
ischemia. However this process is slow, requiring one to
several days.

Therefore the question arises if we can interfere with the
breakdown of adenine nucleotides ? Nucleotides are too polar
to leave the myocardial cell whereas nucleosides and cAMP
can pass the plasma membrane. Two different routes are available for AMP breakdown in the heart : deamination and dephosphorylation. AMP can be deaminated to IMP by AMP deaminase. The alternative pathway is dephosphorylation by 5 nu-
cleotidase. This enzyme dephosphorylates AMP and IMP to form
adenosine or inosine, which both can leave the cell.

This 5 necleotidase is strategically located in the myocardial membranes. ATP and ADP inhibit the enzyme so that it becomes deinhibited under conditions of ischemia. Adenosine can further be converted to inosine by adenosine deaminase in the myocardial cell, in larger vessel walls and in the blood. Adenosine is very vasoactive and produces reactive hyperemia by its action on adenosine receptors on the surface of coronary myocytes. Inosine does not possess vasoactive properties. The adenosine lost from the myocardium is rapidly deaminated to inosine in the endothelium, pericytes and erytrocytes. Inosine is further converted to hypoxanthine by nucleoside phosphorylase. Hypoxanthine is further metabolized in the liver to urate. With the loss of adenosine, the myocardial cell loses its potential for rapid restitution of adenosine nucleotides because the rate of incorporation of adenosine into ATP is much faster than inosine because this has to be degraded to hypoxanthine first.

Adenosine is directly converted to AMP by adeninekinase, located exclusively in the cytoplasm of the myocardial cell.

In an attempt to regenerate ATP after ischemia, ATP and adenosine infusion were unsuccessful. ATP because it cannot penetrate the myocytes and adenosine because its rapid deamination in the blood (10).

The combination of adenosine infusion with adenosine deaminase-blocking agent erythro-9- (2-hydroxy-3-nonyl) adenine hydrochloride (EHNA) however was able to improve myocardial preservation and ATP levels recovered to 88 % of the preischemic values (11).

We found in a series of dog experiments (12) that lidoflazine protects the myocardium during one hour of normothermic global ischemia. Recovery of left ventricular function after 30 minutes of reperfusion is almost complete in contrast with severe low cardiac output in non pretreated animals. Lidoflazine is a potent coronary vasodilatator which potentiates reactive hyperemia.

This suggest an interaction with adenosine.

We know that the uptake of adenosine in red blood cells, which determines the disappearance rate of adenosine, is blocked by lidoflazine. However if lidoflazine influences myocardial ATP levels is not yet investigated.

The protective effects of lidoflazine may also be based on other mechanisms. Lidoflazine is a known calciumchannel blocker and this leads us to another aspect of myocardial ischemia and reperfusion : calcium.

In the normal myocyte, we have a hughe gradient in calcium : $10 - {}^3M$ calcium in the extracellular space compared with $10 - {}^7M$ calcium in the cytosol.

Also intracellular there are gradients in calcium concentration; the sarcoplasmic reticulum can establish calcium concentration ratios of over 3000 between its inner and outer membrane system. Also the mitochondria will easily take calcium up : a fast mitochondrial membrane loading and a slow matrix loading. During ischemia, intracellular concentrations of inorganic phosphate, which is no more incorporated in ADP to form ATP, can increase above a certain level and promote calciumphosphate precipitations (13). This trapping of calcium by phosphate occurs in the sarcoplasmic reticulum,which is permeable for phosphate,and in the mitochondria.

These precipitates may in part be responsible for the early pump failure of the ischemic heart : the availability of calcium for excitation - contraction coupling decreases.

Such changes influence the distribution of calcium, but not the total content.

During reperfusion however, a massive influx of calcium in the cell occurs. This is the consequence of leakage of the cell membranes.

This pathologic influx of calcium after cellmembrane damage, manifested by large calcium precipitates in the mitochondria (Jennings-granules) is largely prevented by lidoflazine (12). For a better understanding of these processes and possible pharmacologic interventions it is necessary to look at the distribution of high energy phosphates in the myocardial cell.

As already mentioned, interruption of blood flow causes an immediate drop in oxygen tension with an halt in aerobic energy production i.e. cessation of oxidative phosphorylation. However, it is remarkable that this goes along with an initial marked decrease in the content of phospocreatine but there is only a modest (10 - 20 %) decrease in ATP content at the same time that myocardial contractility decreases. Creatine phosphate can only provide energy for cell function by transferring high energy phosphate first to ATP.

If this ATP were distributed uniformly throughout the myocardial cell water, ATP concentration would be over 4 mmol/L, a level that saturates contractile proteins and contractile ion pumps. This suggests that only a portion of the cell ATP content is in equilibrium with most or all of the cell phosphocreatine in a discrete compartment.

This ATP seems to be compartmentalized in the cell.

In addition to providing chemical energy for the contractile process and ion pumps, ATP has important effects on the control of myocardial cell function such as regulation of phosphofructokinase, ATP can also promote sodium - calcium exchange. These modulatory actions of ATP require levels which are considerably higher than that needed to saturate the substrate binding sites for contraction.

It is also postulated (14) that aerobically produced ATP may supply energy for contraction whereas glycolytically produced ATP may be linked to membrane electrical activity and the ionic pumps. A submembrane nondiffusible ATP-pool may be supplied preferentially by strategically positioned glycolytic enzymes, especially membrane bound phosphoglyceratekinase. Also cardiac sarcoplasmic reticulum has associated with it a system of glycogenolytic enzymes and because the SR is impermeable to ATP, glycolysis in this organelle may be important in the controle of intracellular calcium ion concentrations. This glycolytically formed ATP may be available for membrane functions. ATP used for contractile functions originates from the mitochondria mainly out of the oxidation of fatty acids. Longchainacyl CoA, the activated form of fatty acids cannot enter the mitochondria by diffusion.

Carnitine, an aminoacid, is needed to form acylcarnitine which can permeate the mitochondrial membrane via the carnitine palmytil CoA transferase (carnitine carrier). Intramitochondrial acyl CoA is further metabolized via betaoxidation and the citric acid cycle.

The produced ATP again cannot diffuse freely through the mitochondrial membrane. A "swing door" mechanism, the ATP translocase system exchanges one molecule ADP for one molecule ATP. This translocase system is a critical link between the energy metabolism of the mitochondrial compartment and that of the cytosol. Accumulation of acylco A in the mitochondria inhibit not only oxydative phosphorylation but also this ATP translocase enzyme.

Ischemia can be reduced by administration of carnitine. Carnitine can combine with activated long chain fatty acids to form acylcarnitine, thus lowering longchain acyl CoA and consequently deinhibiting ATP translocase.

A last aspect concerns subcellular membranes.

Membranes are composed of a phospholipid bilayer. Most phospholipids consist of a glycerol "backbone" in which two fatty acids are esterified to form the nonpolar "tails". The third hydroxyl group is bound to a phosphate containing polar "head" the phosphatide. Ischemic damage to these membranes is due to the effects of amphiphile substances. Amphiphiles are soluble substances which contain both hydrophilic (polar) and hydrophobic (non polar) groups.

At low concentrations in an aqueous medium amphiphiles act as monomers. They incorporate into biological membranes and change the physical properties of the lipid bilayer.

At higher concentrations they act as micelles which have the ability to incorporate membrane lipids into their structure, thereby forming mixed micelles, this detergent like action causes biological membranes to break down, liberating lysophosphatides which are amphiphiles.

The "membrane stabilizing" effect of low concentrations of amphiphiles and the"detergent-like"effect of high concen-

trations represent the biphasic effect of these substances.
Low concentrations of local anesthetics (dicubaïne) reduce
the calcium permeability of the sarcoplasmic reticulum whereas
higher concentrations increase calcium permeability. Three
mechanisms by which incorporation of amphiphilic molecules
into the membrane phospholipids can modify membrane function
are proposed by Katz (15) :
1. membrane expansion
2. calcium displacement
3. annular disruption : the function of membrane proteins
   as receptors, enzymes or channels can be influenced by
   the physical state of the surrounding membrane lipids.

Membrane stabilizing drugs used to prevent ischemic damage
are :
1. local anesthetics (lidocaïne) by membrane expansion and
   calcium displacement.
2. glucocorticosteroïds : hydrocortisone and methyl pred-
   nisolone by stabilizing lysosomal and other cellular
   membranes.
3. Some calcium antagonists : presumably lidoflazine by
   its indirect action on calcium influx. Several phospho-
   lipases may be activated by calcium during ischemia and
   degrade membrane phospholipids.
   The free lysophosphatides exert very detrimental effects
   on membranes : they are able to disrupt the membranes
   further due to their wedge like structure.

It is concluded that pharmacologic interventions bases on
a wide spectrum of metabolic alterations during ischemia may improve tolerance to ischemia of the myocardium. However,
further research in this field is definitely necessary.

REFERENCES

1. KOBAYASHI K. and NEELY J.R.
   Control of maximum rates of glycolysis in rat cardiac muscle.
   Circ. Res. 44 : 166 - 175, 1979

2. BRETSCHNEIDER H.J., HUBNER G., KNOLL D., LOHR B., NORDECLA H.,
   and SPIEKERMANN P.G.
   Myocardial resistance and tolerance to ischemia : physiological and biochemical basis.
   J. Cardiovasc. Surg. 16 : 241 - 260, 1975

3. JUNGE P., HEARSE D.J., BRAINBRIDGE M.
   Myocardial protection during ischemic cardiac arrest.
   J. Thorac Cardiovasc. surg. 73 : 848, 1977

4. FLAMENG W., BORGERS M., DAENEN W. and STALPAERT G.
   Ultrastructural and cytochemical correlates of myocardial
   protection by cardiac hypothermia in man.
   J. Thorac Cardiovasc. surg. 79 : 413, 1980

5. BUCKBERG G.D., BRAZIER J.R., WELSON R.L., GOLDSTEIN C.M.,
   Mc CONNELL D.H. and COOPER N.
   Studies of the effects of hypothermia on regional myocar-
   dial blood flow and metabolism during cardiopulmonary bypass.
   I. The adequately perfused beating, fibrillated and arres-
      ted heart.
   J. Thorac. Cardiovasc. Surg. 73 : 87, 1977

6. MAROKO P.R., KJEKSHUS J.K., and SOBEL B.F.
   Factors influencing infarct size following coronary artery
   occlusion.
   Circulation 43 : 67, 1971

7. WATTS J.A., KOCH C.D. and LA NOUE K.F.
   Effects of Ca^{2+} antagonism on energy metabolism : Ca^{2+} and
   heart function after ischemia.
   Am.J.Physiol. 238 : H 909 - H 916,1980.

8. DA LUZ P.L., MONTIERO DE BARROS L.F., JORGE LEITE, J. PILEGGI
   F. and DECOURT L.V.
   Effect of Verapamil on regional coronary and myocardial
   perfusion during acute coronary occlusion.
   Am. J. Cardiol : 45: 269 - 275,1980

9. VAN DER VUSSE G.J., VAN BELLE H., VAN GERVEN W., KRUGER R.,
   and RENEMAN R.G.
   Acute effect of Fentanyl on hemodynamics and myocardial
   carbohydrate utilization and phosphate release during ischemia.
   Br. J. Anaesth. 51: 927 -935, 1979

10. REIBEL D.K. and ROVETTO M.J.
    Myocardial ATP synthesis and mechanical function following
    oxygen deficiency.
    Am. J. Physiol. 234 (5) : H 620 - H 624, 1978

11. FOKER J.E., EINZIG S. and WANG T.
    Adenosine metabolism and myocardial preservation.
    J. Thorax cardiovasc. Surg. 80 : 506 - 516, 1980

12. FLAMENG W., DAENEN W., BORGERS M., THONE F., XHONNEUX R.,
    VAN DE WATER A. and VAN BELLE H.
    Cardioprotective effects of lidoflazine.
    Circulation (in press)

13. KUBLER W. and KATZ A.
    Mechanism of early "pump" failure of the ischemic heart :
    possible role of adenosine triphosphate depletion and
    inorganic phosphate accumulation.
    A.M.J. Cardiol. 40: 467 - 471, 1977

14. BRICKNELL O.L. and OPIE L.H.
    Effects of substrates on tissue metabolic changes in the
    isolated rat heart during underperfusion and on release of
    lactate dehydrogenase and arrhythmias during reperfusion.
    Circ. Res. 43: 102 - 115, 1978

15. KATZ A.M., and MESINEO F.C.
    Lipid-membrane interactions and the pathogenesis of ischemic
    damage in the myocardium.
    Circ. Res. 48: 1 - 16, 1981

ISOFLURANE

N. TY SMITH, M.D.
E.I. EGER, II, M.D.

INTRODUCTION.

Since it is the only recently developed inhalational anesthetic released, isoflurane is the lone inhalational anesthetic discussed in this symposium on newer agents. Although it is usually compared with other inhalation agents, we shall primarily compare it with the newer intravenous agents. This approach makes particular sense because isoflurane has narrowed or eliminated many of the disadvantages of inhalation agents relative to intravenous agents. Many of our comparisons relate to differences in the general nature of inhalation and intravenous agents. Others are more closely related to properties specific to isoflurane. Because of the great diversity of the intravenous agents, we shall refer to them mainly in general terms, while treating isoflurane much more specifically.

Speed of action. Isoflurane and many of the intravenous agents can rapidly induce anesthesia. Isoflurane's low blood/gas partition coefficient permits a rapid rise in alveolar/inspired concentration (1). However, its mildly pungent odor can limit the rapidity with which the inspired concentration can be increased without producing breathholding or coughing. The speed of induction with intravenous agents may be limited by many factors: chest-wall rigidity (2), hypertonus, excitatory effects, pain on injection, or cardiovascular depression (3). Combinations of intravenous agents can be given to prevent some of these complications. For every problem solved, however, another is often added (4). To avoid these problems we often combine intravenous and inhalation agents for induction.

Although many intravenous agents can be titrated by addition, few can be titrated by subtraction. That is, anesthetic depth can be increased as rapidly or more rapidly with intravenous agents as with isoflurane. However, the effects of most intravenous agents decline at a slower rate than those of isoflurane. This implies an easier control of anesthetic depth with isoflurane. This phenomenon is also important postoperatively. With isoflurane, the chances of prolonged neuromuscular block is minimized (Elimination of isoflurane eliminates the potentiation of relaxant effect--see below). Renarcotization cannot occur. On the other hand, postoperative analgesia may also be limited with isoflurane, and many anesthetists administer a small amount of narcotic intravenously at the end of an inhalation anesthetic to produce postoperative analgesia and smooth the transition from anesthesia to wakefulness.

Biotransformation and toxicity. Biotransformation of isoflurane is minimal in miniature swine (5), Fisher 344 rats (6), mice (7), and man (8). In man, less than 0.2% of the isoflurane taken up can be recovered as urinary metabolites (8). In contrast, 2.4% of enflurane (9) and 15-20% of halothane (10) can be recovered. Most intravenous anesthetics ultimately require biodegradation for their elimination. Isoflurane's minimal metabolism is important because of the frequent association between metabolism of the inhaled agents and their capacity to produce organ toxicity (11). We now assume that inhalation anesthetic agents by themselves are not hepatotoxic, although their metabolites or metabolic intermediates may be (12,13). If this is true, toxicity of anesthetics is directly related to their biodegradation. Isoflurane has two advantages in this regard: it has a low blood/gas partition coefficient and will be available for biodegradation for less time, and it resists biodegradation more than any other inhaled agent (8).

Results from a study in 1975 suggested that isoflurane is a hepatocarcinogen (14). This delayed isoflurane's release for clinical use. Repetition of Corbett's study (15) failed to confirm his results despite the use of larger numbers of animals and of higher and lower doses of isoflurane. Re-examination of the methods used in the original study revealed that inappropriate controls had been used, and bias had not been excluded through a blind examination of control and test specimens. In addition, animals in the first study had been contaminated with potential carcinogens (polybrominated biphenyls). The negative results from the second study are consistent with negative findings for isoflurane from studies of mutagenicity (16,17,18), and it may be concluded that this agent is not a significant carcinogen.

The subject of operating room pollution has been controversial. Isoflurane's resistance to biodegradation strongly suggests that, whatever one's beliefs on the subject, pollution should be a slight or nonexistent problem with this agent. There are, however, no epidemiological data relating to isoflurane. Although intravenous agents alone cannot cause operating room pollution, most of them must be used with nitrous oxide, which of all the inhaled agents is currently the most suspect (19). Since potent agents such as isoflurane do not require the use of nitrous oxide, their employment in oxygen or oxygen-air may decrease or eliminate the risks resulting from atmospheric pollution.

The anesthetic state. In contrast to individual injected anesthetics, isoflurane can produce all of the necessary components of anesthesia (20). Thus, as stated above, isoflurane can be used without nitrous oxide. This is particularly useful when a high inspired concentration of oxygen is required, for example, during thoracotomies, or for patients with severe lung disease. Most intravenous agents depend on nitrous oxide to minimize dose requirements. Although certain intravenous agents can be used without nitrous oxide, the technique is usually reserved for minor surgery or for patients whose postoperative care more routinely requires mechanical ventilation, for example, those undergoing open-heart surgery. The common use of total intravenous anesthesia is in the future.

Although isoflurane given without adjuvants can satisfy all anesthetic requirements, some of the effects of deeper levels of isoflurane may be unnecessary or even undesirable. For example, hypotension may occur before neuromuscular blockade is achieved. Intravenous agents are usually more specifically targeted and are given in combinations aiming to produce a desirable composite effect. Although useful in many cases, such polypharmacy can lead to unanticipated and even undesirable drug interactions. The number of drug interactions increases markedly with the number of drugs given (21).

As with other inhaled agents, it is easier to estimate the depth of anesthesia with isoflurane than with injected agents. The alveolar isoflurane concentration can be predicted with some precision from the delivered concentration. This results from the low blood/gas partition coefficient (1.4) of isoflurane (1). Since the brain partial pressure rapidly equilibrates with that in the alveoli, it is easy to estimate brain concentrations with isoflurane. As a corollary, awareness should be less common with isoflurane. However, isoflurane possesses a far smaller margin of safety than many intravenous agents. The difference approaches two orders of magnitude when isoflurane is compared with some of the newer agents available outside the United States (22).

The electroencephalograph. In anesthetizing concentrations, isoflurane-induced EEG changes appear superficially similar to those of many intravenous agents (Fig. 1a, 1b), with an initial increase in amplitude and decrease in frequency, and progression to burst suppression and ultimately to a flat EEG (23,24,25,26). Both halothane and enflurane produce an EEG which is quantifiable in regards to depth of anesthesia. (27,28) Isoflurane has not been tested enough to indicate the quantifiability of its EEG.

However, the fact that it becomes flat at clinical concentrations suggests that quantification may be difficult at deeper levels. The intravenous agents vary widely in this regard, with diazepam at the difficult end of the spectrum, and the barbiturates at the easy end. Our ability to

176

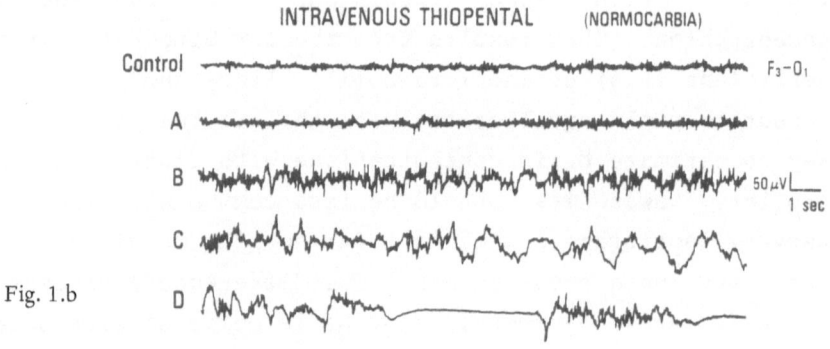

EEG PATTERN IN THE AWAKE STATE
AND DURING ANESTHESIA WITH ISOFLURANE IN OXYGEN

	B. ANESTH. VOLUME	ANESTH. STATE

NORMAL WAKING ACTIVITY (10-14 c.p.s.) — 0.0 — AWAKE

LOW VOLTAGE FAST ACTIVITY (15-20 c.p.s., 20-60 μV) — 0.56 — VERY LIGHT

HIGH VOLTAGE SLOW ACTIVITY (4-6 c.p.s., 40-80 μV) — 0.96 — LIGHT SURGICAL

IRREGULAR SLOW ACTIVITY PATTERN (3-4 c.p.s., 150-200 μV) — 1.78 — MOD. SURGICAL

ALTERNATING ACTIVITY PATTERN (100-250 μV) — 2.20

OCCASIONAL LOW VOLTAGE ACTIVITY — 2.90 — DEEP SURGICAL

Fig. 1.a

INTRAVENOUS THIOPENTAL (NORMOCARBIA)

Control — F_3-O_1

A

B — 50 μV / 1 sec

C

Fig. 1.b

D

FIGURE 1a) Isoflurane in oxygen produces this sequence of electroencephalographic changes as anesthesia deepens. The blood levels ("B. Anesth. Vol %") may be converted to alveolar concentration by dividing by 1.4, the blood/gas partition coefficient. Thus, the 0.96% and 1.78% tracings bracket MAC. From Homi J, et al: A new anesthetic agent--Forane: Preliminary observations in man. Anesth. Analg 51:439-447, 1972. 1b) Electroencephalographic effects of intravenously administered thiopental in man. A, rapid activity at onset of administration. B, spindles of 7-10 Hz. C, slow waves. D, suppressions and intersuppression "bursts." Although different filtering was used, note the similarity to the pattern in Fig. 1a. From Clark DL, Rosner BS: Neurophysiologic effects of general anesthesia. I. The electroencephalogram and sensory evoked responses in man. Anesthesiology 38:564-582, 1973. By kind permission of the author and publishers.

estimate depth of anesthesia by EEG analysis is increasing rapidly. For example, both fentanyl and enflurane produce EEG patterns previously considered too variable to correlate with depth of anesthesia. Recently, however, five EEG levels of fentanyl anesthesia have been reasonably reliably predicted, and results with the spectral-edge frequency and enflurane are very encouraging (28).

Ventilation. Both intravenous and inhalation agents depress ventilation. Isoflurane increases respiratory rate and decreases tidal volume at light levels of anesthesia (29). Deepening anesthesia further decreases tidal volume but does not change respiratory rate. In unstimulated human volunteers, spontaneous ventilation produces a PCO_2 of 50 torr at 1 MAC isoflurane and 65 torr at 1.5 MAC (Fig. 2). The substitution of nitrous oxide for an equivalent amount of isoflurane decreases P_aCO_2 considerably (Fig. 2). The ventilatory response to increased arterial CO_2 is 30% of the awake value at 1 MAC and 14% at 1.5 MAC. Surgical stimulation largely reverses the depression caused by isoflurane (30,31), and mechanical ventilation may not be required to produce a PCO_2 below 50 torr, particularly in the presence of nitrous oxide.

In humans, the ventilatory response to hypoxia is depressed by more than 50% at 1 MAC isoflurane, and further reduced at 1.5 MAC (30). Some of the newer intravenous agents, for example etomidate or midazolam, do not depress (31), or produce only a transient depression of (31), ventilation. In contrast, clinically useful doses of narcotics depress ventilation. This depression is difficult to reverse with surgical stimulation, and it may be prolonged postoperatively.

Circulation. Isoflurane depresses myocardial "contractility" in vitro (32), but not in vivo (33). Anesthetizing doses of most of the newer intravenous agents depress contractility only minimally (31). In unmedicated healthy human volunteers maintained at normal arterial PCO_2 and body temperature, 1 to 2 MAC isoflurane does not alter cardiac output, ballistocardiograph IJ wave amplitude,

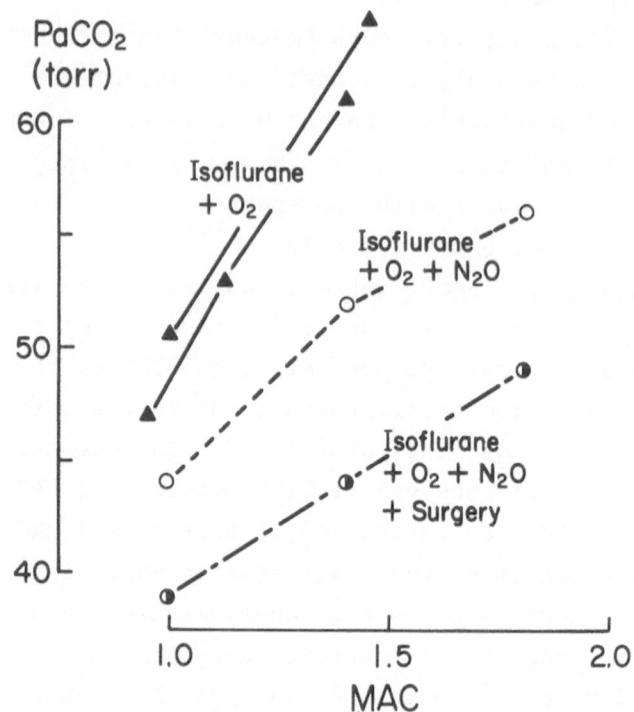

FIGURE 2. The respiratory depressant effect of isoflurane is attenuated by substituting 70% nitrous oxide for an equivalent amount of isoflurane. It is antagonized by surgical stimulation.

ejection time, mean rate of ventricular ejection or pre-ejection period (33) (Fig. 3). Cardiac output is maintained by an increased heart rate which compensates for a moderate reduction of stroke volume. The increase in heart rate with isoflurane results from a greater depression of vagal activity as opposed to sympathetic activity (34). It should be noted that in several thousand patients given isoflurane in a variety of circumstances, the average increase in pulse rate during maintenance was only one to two beats per minute (M Cahalan, JB Forrest, Unpublished Data). In contrast to the increase in pulse rate that may accompany isoflurane anesthesia, bradycardia may follow induction with large doses of many of the opiates (35,36,37,38). The respiratory depression produced by isoflurane increases arterial PCO_2, which alters the cardiovascular response to

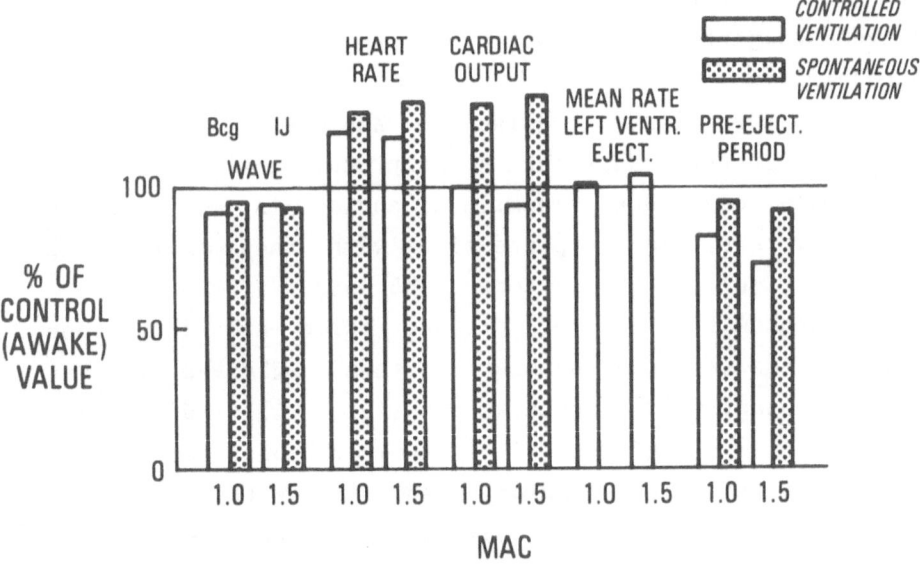

FIGURE 3. A comparison of the circulatory effects of isoflurane during spontaneous vs. controlled ventilation reveals no change in myocardial function (Bcg IJ wave and mean rate left ventricular ejection). Heart rate and cardiac output increase during spontaneous ventilation. From Eger EI, II: Isoflurane: A compendium and reference, 1981. By permission of the author and Ohio Medical Products.

isoflurane during spontaneous ventilation (39). Cardiac output and heart rate exceed awake values, while stroke volume is maintained at awake values (Fig. 3).

Isoflurane could either increase or decrease myocardial oxygen consumption, since the major determinants of myocardial oxygen consumption are heart rate, ventricular wall tension (afterload), and "contractility." On one hand, patients with coronary artery disease may benefit from a decrease in myocardial work (and hence oxygen demand) and maintained or augmented oxygen supply. By producing marked peripheral vasodilation, isoflurane decreases afterload and preload. Unlike other inhalation agents, isoflurane does not increase right atrial pressure (33), and therefore preload. These advantages may be offset by the increase in pulse rate, which, if present, would increase heart work and decrease oxygen delivery. The lack of decrease in contractility also sets isoflurane apart from enflurane and halothane, and isoflurane does not offer the protection to the myocardium that these agents do. Nor, for that matter, do the intravenous agents, which may permit sustained afterload and contractility.

Isoflurane dilates resistance and capacitance vessels (33), while intravenous agents often produce little change or may increase resistance. Thus, hypotension is more common with isoflurane, and hypertension with the intravenous agents, particularly the narcotics (35,36,37).

The concomitant use of nitrous oxide and isoflurane produces less arterial hypotension than isoflurane alone at equivalent anesthetic concentrations (40). This difference results from a difference in systemic vascular resistance. The effect of nitrous oxide when used with isoflurane contrasts with its detrimental effects when used with narcotics. Nitrous oxide added to a narcotic anesthetic decreases arterial pressure and cardiac output (41,42,43,44), and the effect can be profound in ill patients.

In dogs, propranolol does not alter the impact of isoflurane on blood pressure (Fig. 4) or cardiac output (45). Their data imply that isoflurane can probably be given safely in the presence of therapeutic levels of beta-adrenergic blockade.

Arterial pressure is easier to control with isoflurane, and can often be modulated to meet surgical requirements. This means that intravenous vasodilating agents are rarely required with isoflurane. This would appear to be an advantage of this agent, since the use of vasodilators such as sodium nitroprusside poses many risks and exacts many prices. A separate intravenous line, preferably central, should be used to infuse nitroprusside. Constant attention is required for infusing nitroprusside, attention which may have to be diverted from other areas of patient care. Disaster can occur if the line is inadvertently flushed. Even with undivided attention, physician and nurse anesthetists may infuse nitroprusside in a poor or even dangerous manner (47).

Isoflurane is the only currently available anesthetic--inhaled or intravenous--that markedly increases

ARTERIAL PRESSURE
(torr)

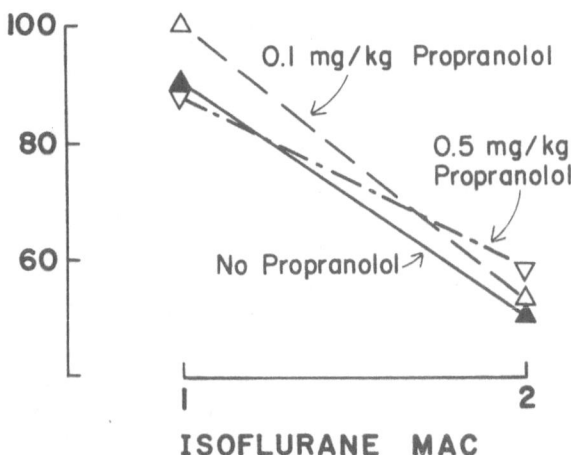

FIGURE 4. The effects of 1 and 2 MAC isoflurane on mean systemic arterial pressure were measured before and after administration of 0.1 and 0.5 mg/kg of propranolol. No enhancement of the depressant effect of isoflurane occurred. From Eger EI, II: Isoflurane: A compendium and reference, 1981. By permission of the author and Ohio Medical Products.

muscle blood flow (33). This increase in muscle blood flow can be either useful or disadvantageous. It may accelerate the onset or elimination of the effects of muscle relaxants. In patients undergoing cardiopulmonary bypass, the increased muscle blood flow may produce a more rapid equilibration between muscle and core temperatures and prevent profound falls in the latter following bypass. On the other hand, the increase in flow is wasted nutritionally, and it increases cardiac work.

Light levels of isoflurane (e. g., 0.6-1.1 MAC) do not change cerebral blood flow (Fig. 5) (48). Higher concentrations (1.6 MAC) increase cerebral blood flow (in normotensive, eucapnic volunteers) and intracranial pressure (48). Enflurane causes comparable, while halothane causes greater, increases in flow and pressure. Intracranial pressure may be decreased more readily with mild hyperventilation during isoflurane than during halothane

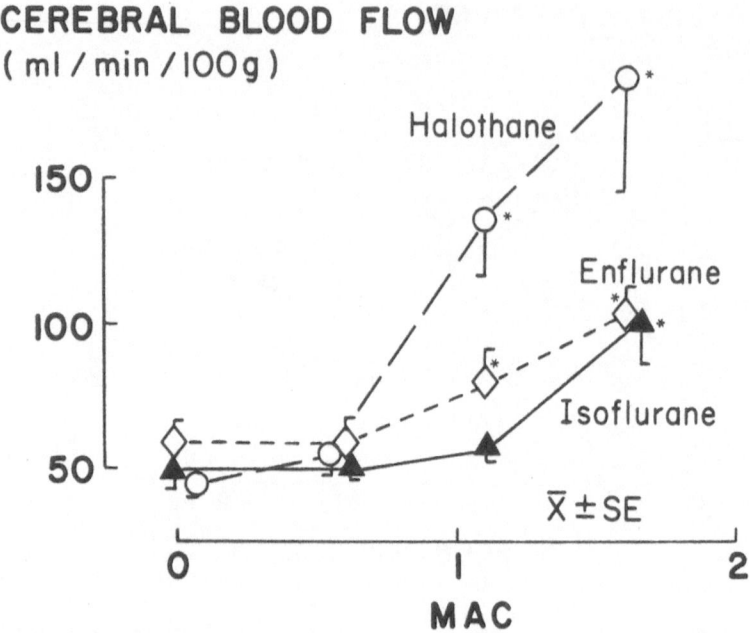

CEREBRAL BLOOD FLOW
(ml / min / 100g)

FIGURE 5. Cerebral blood flow in healthy volunteer subjects during conditions of normotension and normocarbia. Flow increased at light levels of enflurane and halothane anesthesia, but did not increase at the same levels of isoflurane. From Eger EI,II: Isoflurane: A compendium and reference, 1981. By permission of the author and Ohio Medical Products.

anesthesia (49). Except for ketamine, which increases flow (50), the intravenous agents either do not change cerebral blood flow (e.g., narcotics, assuming ventilation is adequately maintained) or may actually decrease it (thiopental, lidocaine, or althesin) (51). The barbiturates are often used to reduce cerebral blood flow and intracranial pressure. Isoflurane and other inhalation agents do not limit, and may increase, the extent of cerebral edema induced by trauma (52). Conversely, pentobarbital, or fentanyl and droperidol (Innovar) do protect against post-traumatic development of edema (Fig. 6) (52).

Neither isoflurane nor the injected agents increase the incidence of ventricular dysrhythmias (53,54). Neither isoflurane nor the intravenous agents sensitize the

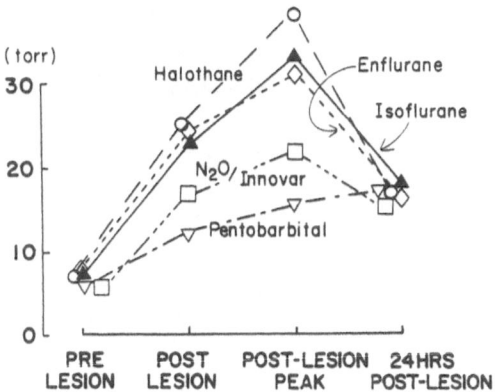

INTRACRANIAL PRESSURE AFTER
CRYOGENIC LESION

FIGURE 6. Small areas of dog cerebral cortex were frozen during halothane anesthesia. Light levels of anesthesia were maintained thereafter with one of the indicated anesthetics. Systemic blood pressure was sustained above 90 torr with phenylephrine. Greater increases in intracranial pressure were associated with volatile anesthetics than with injected agents. From Eger EI, II: Isoflurane: A compendium and reference, 1981. By permission of the author and Ohio Medical Products.

myocardium to the dysrhythmogenic effect of epinephrine (55,56,57). This is another area in which isoflurane has narrowed the difference between inhalation and intravenous agents.

Neuromuscular blockade. The modern potent inhaled anesthetics, such as isoflurane (53,54), can provide relaxation sufficient for any surgical procedure. This characteristic sets them apart from the predominantly narcotic anesthetic, which produces no relaxation and may with some agents be associated with chest wall rigidity (2). The relaxation that attends the use of agents such as isoflurane may make their application particularly valuable in patients suffering from myesthenia gravis, or from liver or kidney impairment, since the anesthetist may prefer not to use muscle relaxants in such patients. However, to achieve profound relaxation with isoflurane alone may require higher concentrations than the patient can tolerate and hence may

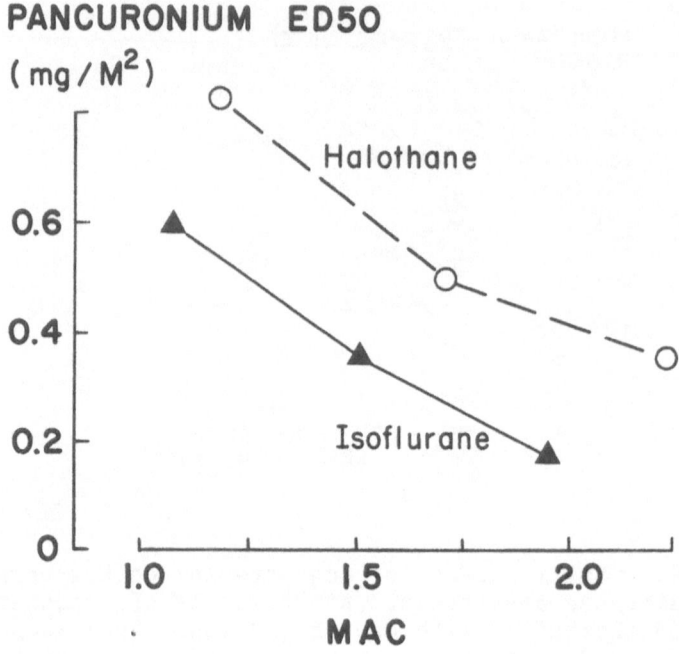

FIGURE 7. The dose of pancuronium required to decrease twitch height by 50% was determined in patients. At any given MAC multiple, isoflurane produced a greater potentiation of pancuronium than did halothane. Deeper levels of either anesthetic increased the potentiation. From Eger EI, II: Isoflurane: A compendium and reference, 1981. By permission of the author and Ohio Medical Products.

lead to the use of muscle relaxants.

In contrast to the intravenous agents, isoflurane markedly potentiates the effects of non-depolarizing neuromuscular blocking agents (58,59) and does so in a dose related fashion (Fig. 7) (60). Consequently, less relaxant is required with isoflurane. More importantly, the neuromuscular block produced by a small amount of muscle relaxant can be titrated, that is rapidly increased or decreased at will, simply by increasing or decreasing the concentration of isoflurane. The rapid removal of the anesthetic agent itself hastens reversal of neuromuscular blockade. Thus, prolonged neuromuscular blockade should be much less common after isoflurane than after the intravenous agents (61).

Malignant hyperthermia. Although no case of malignant hyperthermia has been reported to have occurred during an isoflurane anesthetic, animal studies indicate that isoflurane may precipitate malignant hyperthermia in susceptible patients. Studies in frog sartorius muscle (62), Poland China swine (63), and human skeletal muscle (64) indicate that isoflurane is as effective an initiator of malignant hyperthemia as enflurane. Thus, in susceptible patients it is probably better to use certain intravenous agents, such as Innovar, diazepam, althesin, barbiturates, or narcotics (65). Whatever intravenous agent is used, prophylactic dantrolene is necessary (61).

Nausea and vomiting. Narcotics may stimulate the chemoreceptor trigger zone and cause contraction of smooth muscle. These effects can produce nausea and vomiting. It has not been demonstrated that isoflurane stimulates the chemoreceptor trigger zone and contracts smooth muscle. Nausea and vomiting can be so distressing with some intravenous agents that other agents are often routinely administered for prevention.

Obstetrical anesthesia and analgesia. Isoflurane produces a significant dose-related depression of contractility of human uterine muscle in vitro (66). Like halothane, isoflurane anesthesia increases uterine bleeding during therapeutic suction abortion and, therefore, is not suitable for this procedure (67,68).

Not enough experience is available with isoflurane to assess its proper role in obstetrics. Animal experiments suggest that uterine blood flow and fetal oxygenation are well sustained at 1 or 1.5 MAC but may be compromized at 2 MAC (69). Although hypoxia and acidosis do not occur, the direct narcotizing effect of isoflurane may produce neonatal depression at 1 and 1.5 MAC. Isoflurane may compare well with nitrous oxide for analgesia during childbirth. Isoflurane has the advantage of rapid excretion if the newborn infant is ventilated adequately. In any case, the same need for light anesthesia applies equally to isoflurane and the intravenous agents. The endeavor to maintain light levels of anesthesia has led to a higher incidence of awareness during caesarean sections than during any other operative procedure. This awareness is probably less likely with the administration of potent inhalation agents than with a nitrous oxide-narcotic anesthetic. In the authors' opinion, regional anesthesia remains the anesthesia of choice for most obstetrical procedures.

Pediatric anesthesia. The low blood/gas partition coefficient and the theoretically rapid induction with isoflurane would seem to be an advantage in pediatric anesthesia, particularly in the outpatient setting. However, isoflurane's mildly pungent odor and airway irritation may counterbalance this advantage. Nevertheless, the rapidity with which isoflurane is excreted, and the consequently rapid recovery, make isoflurane ideal in the outpatient area.

Endocrine changes. Blood glucose is elevated during isoflurane anesthesia and surgery in man (70,71) perhaps because of a release of growth hormone. (71) Plasma insulin levels do not increase significantly (71,72,73). Surgery during isoflurane anesthesia increases circulating thyroxine levels in man (71,72).

As with other potent agents, isoflurane may decrease intraocular pressure. Such an effect may be advantageous in ophthalmic surgery. Thiopental, ketamine, Innovar, etomidate, diazepam, and midazolam all reduce intraocular pressure, with reductions ranging from 1.4 to 7.0 torr (74). None of these drugs, however, will protect against the increase in intraocular pressure seen following the administration of succinylcholine and the performance of endotracheal intubation. It is not known whether isoflurane offers such protection.

Summary. With the advent of isoflurane, the gap between inhalation and intravenous agents has narrowed. The advantageous similarities include relative rapidity of induction, ease of deepening the level during maintenance, essentially no long-term toxicity, superficially similar EEG's, minimal myocardial depression in vivo, and lack of myocardial sensitization to epinephrine. Disadvantageous similarities include depression of ventilation and possible lack of protection against myocardial ischemia. There remain, however, important differences. Some differences favor isoflurane; some favor the intravenous agents. Included in the former are: rapid emergence; greater versatility; greater completeness of anesthesia, including more nearly certain amnesia; no necessity for use with nitrous oxide; easier estimation of depth; ease of modulating blood pressure; and the production and potentiation of neuromuscular blockade. The relative disadvantages of isoflurane concern: shorter postoperative analgesia; an increase in heart rate; increased muscle and cerebral blood flow; a lack of protection against traumatically induced cerebral edema; potential precipitation of malignant hyperthemia; induction of uterine relaxation; and increased surgical uterine bleeding. Thus, the perfect anesthetic agent is still not available, and both isoflurane and the intravenous agents have their place in the modern practice of anesthesia. An interesting possibility, which remains to be explored, is that a combination of the two approaches may produce a result closer to the ideal than either alone.

REFERENCES

1. Cromwell TH, Eger EI II, Stevens WC, Dolan WM: Forane uptake, excretion, and blood solubility in man. Anesthesiology 35:401-408, 1971.
2. Hug CC, Jr.: What is the role of narcotic analgesics in anesthesia? American Society of Anesthesiologists, Refresher Course Lecture No. 138, 1980, p.2.
3. Dundee JW: The ideal intravenous anesthetic(s), in Trends in Intravenous Anesthesia, Aldrete JA, Stanley TH (eds), Miami, Symposia Specialists Inc., 1980, p 127-144.
4. Zacharias M: Etomidate, in Trends in Intravenous Anesthesia, Aldrete JA, Stanley TH (eds), Miami, Symposia Specialists, Inc., 1980, p 173-188.
5. Halsey MJ, Sawyer DC, Eger EI II, et al: Hepatic metabolism of halothane, methoxyflurane, cyclopropane, Ethrane and Forane in miniature swine. Anesthesiology 35:43-47, 1971.
6. Van Dyke R: Biotransformation of volatile anaesthetics with special emphasis on the role of metabolism in the

188

toxicity of anaesthetics. Can Anaesth Soc J 20:21-33, 1973.

7. Fiserova-Bergerova V: Changes of fluoride content in bone. Anesthesiology 38:345-351, 1973.

8. Holaday DA, Fiserova-Bergerova V, Latto IP, et al: Resistance of isoflurane biotransformation in man. Anesthesiology 43:325-332, 1975.

9. Chase RE, Holaday DA, Fiserova-Bergerov V, et al: The biotransformation of Ethrane in man. Anesthesiology 35:252-267, 1971.

10. Rehder K, Forbes J, Alter H, et al: Halothane biotransformation in man: A quantitative study. Anesthesiology 28:711-715, 1967.

11. Cohen EN, Van Dyke RA: Metabolism of volatile anesthesia: Implications for toxicity. Reading, Massachusetts, Addison-Wesley, 1977.

12. Brown BR, Jr.: Anesthetic hepatic toxicity: A scientific problem? International Anesthesia Research Society Refresher Course, 1979.

13. Zumbiel MA, Fiserova-Bergerova V, Malinin TI, Holaday DA: Glutathione depletion following inhalation anesthesia. Anesthesiology 49:102-108, 1978.

14. Corbett TH: Cancer and congenital anomalies associated with anesthetics. Ann NY Acad Sci 271:58-66, 1976.

15. Eger EI II, White AE, Brown CL, Biava CG, Corbett TH, Stevens WC: A test of the carcinogenicity of enflurane, isoflurane, halothane, methoxyflurane, and nitrous oxide in mice. Anesth Analg 57:678-694, 1978.

16. Baden JM, Kelley M, Wharton RS, et al: Mutagenicity of halogenated ether anesthetics. Anesthesiology 46:346-350, 1977.

17. Waskell L: A study of the mutagenicity of anesthetics and their metabolites. Mutat. Res. 57:141-153, 1978.

18. White AE, Takehisa S, Eger EI II, et al: Sister chromatid exchanges induced by inhaled anesthetics. Anesthesiology 50:426-430, 1979.

19. Cohen EN, Brown BW, Bruce DL, et al: A survey of anesthetic health hazards among dentists. JADA 90:1291-1296, 1975.

20. Eger EI II: Isoflurane (Forane), A Compendium and Reference, Airco Inc., 1981.

21. Smith N Ty: Drug interactions: Challenge and opportunity, in Drug Interactions in Anesthesia, Smith N Ty, Miller RD, Corbascio AN (eds), Philadelphia, Lea and Febiger, 1981, p 1-9.

22. Investigator's Brochure for Sufentanil. Janssen Pharmaceutica, 1980.

23. Stockard J, Bickford R: The neurophysiology of anaesthesia. In: A Basis and Practice of Neuroanaesthesia, Gordon E (ed), Amsterdam, Excerpta Medica 1975, p 3-46.

24. Eger EI II, Stevens WC, Cromwell TH: The electroencephalogram in man anesthetized with Forane. Anesthesiology 35:504-508, 1971.

25. Clark DL, Hosick EC, Adam N, Castro AD, Rosner BS, Neigh JL: Neural effects of isoflurane (Forane) in man. Anesthesiology 39:261-270, 1973.

26. Clark DL, Rosner BS: Neurophysiologic effects of general anesthetics: I. The electroencephalogram and sensory evoked responses in man. Anesthesiology 38:564-582, 1973.

27. Smith NT, Rampil IJ, Sasse FG, et al: EEG during rapidly changing halotha or enflurane. Anesthesiology 51:S4, 1979.

28. Rampil IF, Sasse FJ, Smith N, Ty et al: Spectral edge frequency - A new correlate of anesthetic depth (Abstract), Anesthesiology 53: 3S, p. S12, 1980.

29. Fourcade HE, Stevens WC, Larson CP, et al: The ventilatory effects of Forane, a new inhaled anesthetic. Anesthesiology 35:26-31, 1971.

30. Hirshman CA, McCullough RE, Cohen PG, Weil JV: Depression of hypoxic ventilatory response by halothane, enflurane, and isoflurane in dogs. Br J Anaesth 49:957, 1977.

31. Stanley TH: Pharmacology of intravenous non-narcotic anesthetic (excluding ketamine), American Society of Anesthesiologists Refresher Course Lecture No. 235, p 1-11.

32. Kemmotsu O, Hashimoto Y, Shimosato S: Inotropic effects of isoflurane on mechanics of contraction in isolated cat papillary muscles from normal and failing hearts. Anesthsiolology 39:470-477, 1973.

33. Stevens WC, Cromwell TH, Halsey MH, et al: The cardiovascular effects of a new inhalation anesthetic, Forane, in human volunteers at constant arterial carbon dioxide tension. Anesthesiology 35:3-16, 1971.

34. Skovsted P, Sapthavichaikul S: The effects of isoflurane on arterial pressure, pulse rate, autonomic nervous activity and barostatic reflexes. Can. Anaesth Soc J 24:304-314, 1977.

35. Estafanous FG, Tarazi RC, Viljoen JF, et al: Systemic hypertension following myocardial revascularization. American Heart Journal 85:732-738, 1973.

36. Arens JF, Benbow BP, Ochsner JL: Morphine anesthesia for aorto-coronary bypass procedures. Anesth Analg 51:901-907, 1972.

37. Lowenstein E: Morphine "Anesthesia" - A Perspective, Anesthesiology 35:563-565, 1971.

38. Drew JH, Dripps RD, Comroe JH: Clinical studies on morphine, II. Effect of morphine upon the circulation of man and upon the circulatory and respiratory responses to tilting. Anesthesiology 7:44-61, 1946.

39. Cromwell TH, Stevens WC, Eger EI II, et al: The cardiovascular effects of compound 469 (Forane) during sponaneous ventilation and CO_2 challenge in man. Anesthesiology 35:17-25, 1971.

40. Dolan WM, Stevens WC, Eger EI II, et al: The cardiovascular and respiratory effects of isoflurane nitrous oxide anesthesia. Can Anaesth Soc J 21:557-568, 1974.

41. McDermott R., Stanley TH: The cardiovascular effects of low concentrations of nitrous oxide during morphine anesthesia. Anesthesiology 41:89-91, 1974.

42. Stanley TH, Liu WS: Cardiovascular effects of meperidine-N_2O anesthesia before and after pancuronium. Anesth Analg. 56:836-841, 1977.
43. Stanley TH, Bidwai AV, Lunn JK, et al: Cardiovascular effects of nitrous oxide during meperidine infusion in the dog. Anesth Analg 56:836-841, 1977.
44. Dobkin AB, Pielock PA, Iserael JS, et al: Circulatory and metabolic effects of Innovar Fentanyl-Nitrous oxide anesthesia for major abdominal surgery in man. Anesth Analg 49:261-267, 1970.
45. Philbin DM, Lowenstein E: Hemodynamic consequences of the combination of isoflurane anesthesia (1 MAC) and beta-adrenergic blockade in the dog. Anestheslogy 42:567-573, 1975.
46. Philbin DM, Lowenstein E: Lack of **beta**-adrenergic activity of isoflurane in the dog: a comparison of circulatory effects of halothane and isoflurane after propranolol administration. Br J Anaesth 48:1165-1170, 1976.
47. Smith N Ty, Flick JT, Quinn M: A controller for the automatic infusion of Na nitroprusside. Does it perform as well as the anesthetist? Abstracts of Scientific Papers, Annual Meeting ASA, 691-692, 1977.
48. Murphy FL, Kennell EM, Johnstone RE, et al: The effects of enflurane, isoflurane and halothane on cerebral blood flow and metabolism in man. Abstracts of Scientific Papers, American Society of Anesthesiologists Annual Meeting:61-21, 1974.
49. Adams RW, Cucchiara RF, Gronert GA, et al: Isoflurane and cerebrospinal fluid pressure in neurosurgical patients. Anesthesiology 54:97-99, 1981.
50. Takeshita H, Okuda Y, Sari A: The effects of ketamine on cerebral circulation and metabolism in man, Anesthesiology 36: 69-75.
51. Shapiro HM: Intracranial hypertension. Therapeutic and anesthetic considerations. Anesthesiology 43:445-471, 1975.
52. Smith AL, Marque JJ: Anesthetics and cerebral edema. Anesthesiology 45:64-72, 1976.
53. Pauca AL, Dripps RD: Clinical experience with isoflurane (Forane), Br J Anaesth 45:697-703, 1973.
54. Raj PP, Todd MJ, Jenkins MT: Clinical comparison of isoflurane and halothane anesthetics. South Med J 69:1128-1132, 1976.
55. Joas TA and Stevens WC: Comparison of the arrhythmic doses of epinephrine during Forane, halothane and fluroxene anesthesia in dogs. Anesthesiology 35:48-53, 1971.
56. Tucker WK, Rackstein AD, Munson ES: Comparison of arrhythmic doses of adrenaline, metaraminol, ephedrine and phenylephrine during isoflurane anesthesia in dogs. Br J Anaesth 46:392-396, 1974.
57. Johnston RR, Eger EI II, Wilson C: A comparative interaction of epinephrine with enflurane, isoflurane and halothane in man. Anesth Analg 55:709-712, 1976.

58. Miller RD, Way WL, Dolan WM, Stevens WC, Eger EI II: Comparative neuromuscular effects of pancuronium, gallamine, and succinylcholine during Forane and halothane anesthesia in man. Anesthesiology 35:509-514, 1971.

59. Vitez TS, Miller RD, Eger EI II, et al: Comparison in vitro of isoflurane and halothane potentiation of d-tubocurarine and succinylcholine neuromuscular blockades. Anesthesiology 41:53-56, 1974.

60. Miller RD, Way WL, Dolan WM, Stevens WC, Eger EI II: The dependence of pancuronium- and d-tubocurarine-induced muscle blockades on alveolar concentrations of halothane and Forane. Anesthesiology 37:537-581, 1972.

61. Ohta Y, Nagashima H, Lofrumento R, Foldes FF: Halothane-isoflurane-relaxant interactions in vivo. Anesthsiology 53:S265, 1980.

62. Reed SB, Strobel GE: An in-vitro model of malignant hyperthermia; differential effects of inhalation anesthetics on caffeine-induced muscle contractures. Anesthesiology 48:254-259, 1978.

63. Murphy FL Jr., Nelson TE, Strobel GE, Jones EW: A comparison of halothane, isoflurane, enflurane and fluroxene in triggering malignant hyperthermia in susceptible swine. Abstacts of Scientific Papers. Am Soc Anesth Annual Meeting , 181-182, 1973.

64. Britt BA, Endrenyi L, Frodis W, et al: Comparison of effects of several inhalation anesthetics on caffeine-induced contractures of normal and malignant hyperthermic skeletal muscle. Can Anaesth Soc J 24:12-15, 1980.

65. Miller J, Lee C: Muscle diseases, in **Anesthesia and Unusual Diseases**, Katz J, Benumof J (eds), Philadelphia, W.B. Saunders, 1981, p. 549.

66. Munson ES, Embro WJ: Enflurane, isoflurane and halothane and isolated human uterine muscle. Anesthesiology 46:11-14, 1977.

67. Cullen BF, Margolis AJ, Eger EI II: The effects of anesthesia and pulmonary ventilation on blood loss during elective therapeutic abortion. Anesthesiology 32:108-113, 1970.

68. Dolan WM, Eger I II, Margolis AJ: Forane increases bleeding in therapeutic suction abortion. Anesthesiology 36:96-97, 1972.

69. Palahniuk RJ, Shnider SM, Eger EI II: Pregnancy decreases the requirement for inhaled anesthetic agents. Anesthesiology 41:82-83, 1974.

70. Stevens WC, Eger EI II, Joas TA, et al: Comparative toxicity of isoflurane, halothane, fluroxene and diethyl ether in human volunteers. Can Anaesth Soc J 20:357-368, 1973.

71. Oyama T, Latto P, Holaday DA: Effect of isoflurane anaesthesia and surgery on carbohydrate metabolism and plasma cortisol levels in man. Can Anesth Soc J 22:696-702, 1975.

72. Oyama T, Latto P, Holaday DA, Chang H: Effect of isoflurane anaesthesia and surgery on thyroid function in man. Can Anaesth So J 22:474-477, 1975.
73. Dobkin AB, Byles PH, Africa BF, Levy AA: Enflurane (Ethrane) and isoflurane (Forane): a comparison with nine general anaesthetics administered with passive hyperventilation. Can Anaesth Soc J 23:5505-515, 1976.
74. Fragen RJ, Hauch TH: The effect of midazolam maleate and diazepam on intraocular pressure in adults. In: Trends in Intravenous Anesthesia, Aldrete JA, Stanley TH (eds), Miami, Symposia Specialists, 1980.

NEW NEUROMUSCULAR BLOCKING AGENTS

S.A.FELDMAN

At present 3 non-depolarizing neuromuscular blocking drugs account for
85 per cent of all the agents used for producing prolonged paralysis, they
are pancuronium, tubocurarine, and alcuronium. Although these agents
have proved to be amongst the least toxic and least dangerous drugs used
in anaesthesia all have potential disadvantages. All cause changes in cardiovascular function - pancuronium causes vagal block[1,2,3] and depression
of non-adrenaline reuptake[4,5], which may result in tachycardia and hypertension - together these two effects increase the rate pressure product
and cardiac work. Tubocurarine releases histamine and may produce hypotension, as indeed may alcuronium. Pancuronium and alcuronium are very cumulative drugs and their block may be difficult to reverse, especially
in the presence of a low glomerular filtration rate. Although tubocurarine causes less instances of reversal difficulties it is the longest acting drug of the three and so least suitable for shorter operations.
It is against this background that the new neuromuscular blocking agents
must be viewed. To be clinically succesful they must have a significantly better pharmacological profile. Savarese and Kitz[6] in 1975 declared
that in their opinion there was a need for 3 different drugs, each with
different pharmacokinetic profiles.
1. An ultrashort acting non-depolarizing drug to replace suxamethonium
2. An intermediate duration drug
3. A long acting drug but with rapid recovery from full block
It was predicted by Feldman[7] that it was unlikely that a non-depolarizing drug of a suxamethonium like duration would be produced, due to the
differing pharmacodynamic characters of depolarizing and non-depolarizing
agents. Indeed it was suggested that it would be more

feasible to seek for a non-depolarizing drug that was moderately long in duration for which the plasma clearance was rapid, thus allowing easy, safe and complete reversal from within 5 - 10 minutes of administration. Such a drug, it was predicted, would have the great advantage of being non-cumulative upon successive dose administration. This has proved to be the case with the new generation of relaxants.

In addition to the pharmacological profiles a new drug must fulfil other considerations -

1. Specificity of action at the neuromuscular junction

2. Ease and convenience in use

Both of these criteria are met by the new generation of non-depolarizing relaxants.

There are 3 new non-depolarizing neuromuscular blocking agents at present under study. They are the steroid ORG NC45 (Norcuron), atracurium and the steroid pipercurium (Ardnan). The first 2 drugs are much shorter in duration of action than pipercurium. As yet pipercurium has not been widely used in clinical patients in the West and although we await the results of trials with interest we have insufficient evidence with which to compare its properties with atracurium and ORG NC45.

Atracurium

This drug was synthesised by Stenlake and co-workers at the University of Strathclyde and its pharmacological properties investigated by Hughes and Payne [8,9]. As yet the results of multicentered trials in patients have not been published and our knowledge of its action in humans is more limited than with ORG NC45. The drug appears to have some very attractive features -

1. No cardiovascular changes in up to 15 times a paralytic dose in animals (Fig. 1)

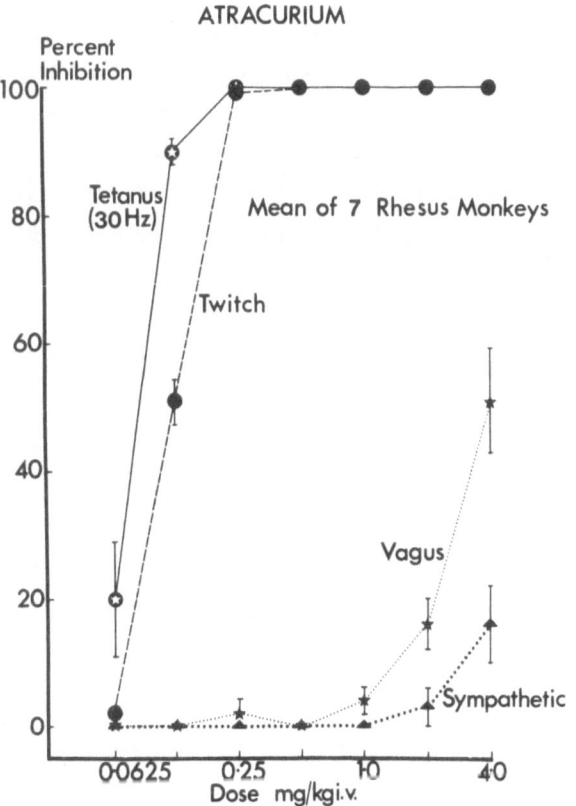

Fig. 1

2.   A lack of cumulative effect in repeated doses given at 10 - 20 per cent recovery.

3.   No prolongation of action in animals following renal pedicle ligation or elimination of hepatic distribution, suggesting biotransformation as the principal means of elimination of the drug.

The dose required to abolish the twitch response is about 300 μg/kg and intubation is said to be possible after 2 minutes with this dose. However, it is suggested that twice this dose, 600 μg/kg, produces more satisfactory clinical block and more useful intubation conditions. With this dose there is usually a period of complete twitch suppression followed by a rapid recovery of full twitch response. The recovery index (25 - 75 per cent recovery time) is in the order of 10 minutes. Reversal with neostigmine after 5 minutes is easily achieved.

This drug is a short acting non-depolarizing muscle relaxant with a high specificity of action. Its mode of elimination in the blood is uncertain, although 2 processes have been shown to occur - Fig. 2.

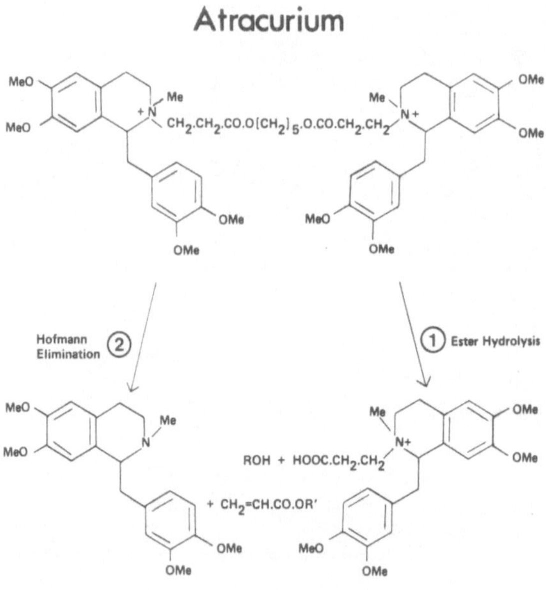

Atracurium

Fig. 2

The Hofmann elimination pathway with the breaking of the C - N linkage and spontaneous ester hydrolysis (not affected by cholinesterase) has in vitro half life of 26 minutes. This by itself would be insufficient to account for the brevity of action of the drug although it is possible that pH changes may accelerate this process.

Although more information is needed about the pharmacokinetics of this drug and its pharmacology in man, initial results suggest that this drug offers substantial advantages over other drugs presently available.

ORG NC45 (Norcuron)

Much more information is available about this agent [10, 11, 12, 13]. This monoquaternary analague of pancuronium was synthesised by David Savage in the Organon laboratories in Strathclyde. Because of the lack of the quaternerizing methyl group at the 2 position, this 2β nitrogen atom destabilises the 3 acetyl group at pH 7. It is therefore necessary to reconstitute the drug from powder using a buffer solution. In spite of this in vitro instability the reconstituted drug does not appear to spontaneously revert to the 3 hydroxy-derivitive in vivo. This metabolite is present in the urine and bile of patients receiving the drug. However, it is likely that this is the result of biotransformation as with pancuronium. ORG NC45 is taken up more readily by the liver than pancuronium which reflects its great lipophillicity. The majority of the drug appears to be excreted in the urine. Details of the pharmacokinetics of this drug are still unpublished although Agoston[14] in a personal communication has indicated that although they do not differ greatly from tubocurarine and pancuronium in their α and β distribution volumes. ORG NC45 is largely excreted unchanged in the urine and bile, biotransformation accounting for less than 2 per cent of the recovered drug. However, larger amounts of the drug can be sequestrated to inactive binding sites. This might explain the relatively small prolongation of action in patients with renal failure (32 per cent compared with 80 per cent for pancuronium).

ORG NC45 (Norcuron) is a short acting non-depolarizing relaxant with little or no cumulative properties. In a well controlled study, Barnes [15] has demonstrated an absence of effect on the heart rate and blood pressure with this drug in a dose of 0.12 mg/Kg. Up to 20 times the paralytic dose has been administered to animals without changes in cardiac parameters.

Like atracurium, ORG NC45 is a short acting neuromuscular blocking agent, devoid of cardiovascular effects in clinical doses. In our experience of over 80 patients we have found it to be predictable in its duration of action in all but two normal individuals. It is virtually non-cumulative on repeated injections - Fig 3.

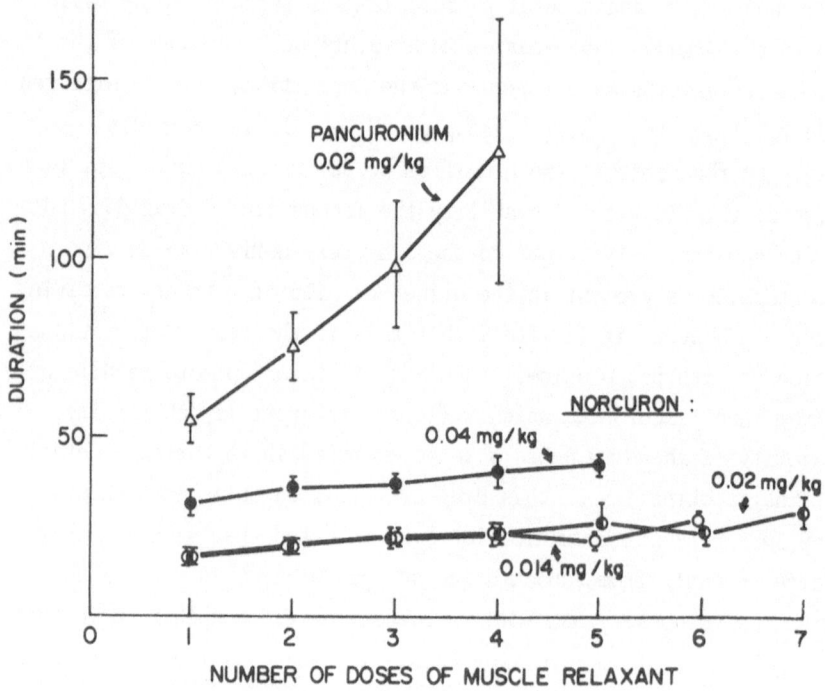

Fig. 3

although some prolongation of the recovery index does occur after 2 - 3 hours of use. Unlike other workers we have not found it significantly better than pancuronium when used for tracheal intubation. In a well controlled study of intubating conditions using 0.10 mg/Kg and 0.15 mg/ Kg Harrison and Feldman [16] found intubation possible at 2 minutes although even at the higher dose range some patients reacted to the intubation. All patients to whom 0.2 mg/Kg were administered were easily intubated with perfect conditions at 90 seconds.

It remains to decide how best to use these new drugs. Because of their short duration of action, their non-cumulative properties and their lack of side effects in doses many times that required for paralysis one of 3 techniques might be suitable for their use -

1.   Administration in frequently repeated small doses

2.   Continuous infusion

3.   Administration as a bolus in multiples of the paralytic dose on the assumption that there is a relationship between the log of the dose and duration of action in normal individuals.

1.   Frequently repeated small doses. Provided an initial dose of 0.1 mg/Kg of ORG NC45 is administered subsequent top up doses of 0.4 to 0.5 mg/Kg will provide relaxation for about 20 - 25 minutes. Fig. 4 is a representation of one such administration during the course of which gentamycin 80 mgs was administered causing a prolongation of block and recovery index.

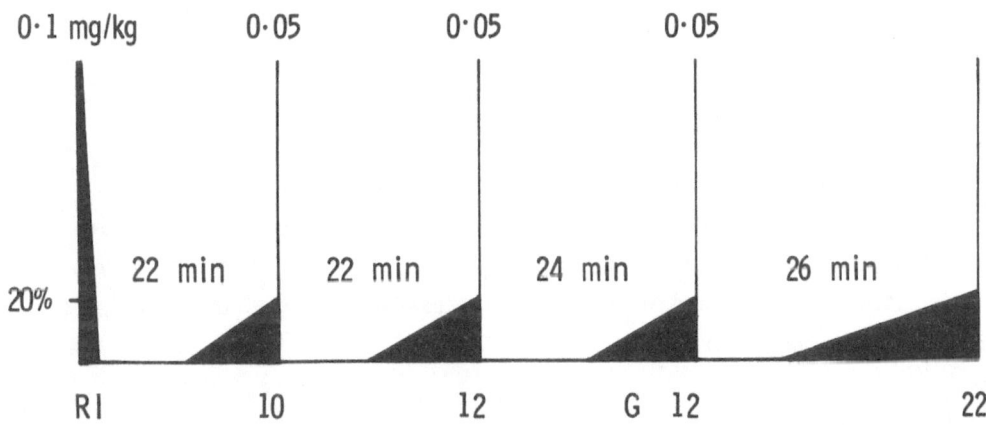

Fig. 4

2. Following an initial dose of 0.05mg/Kg continuous infusion of the drug whilst monitoring the twitch response can be used. This produces reasonable relaxation.Between 0.08 to 0.10 mg/Kg/hr has been required for adequate surgical relaxation - Fig. 5 is a representation of a typical infusion twitch response record.

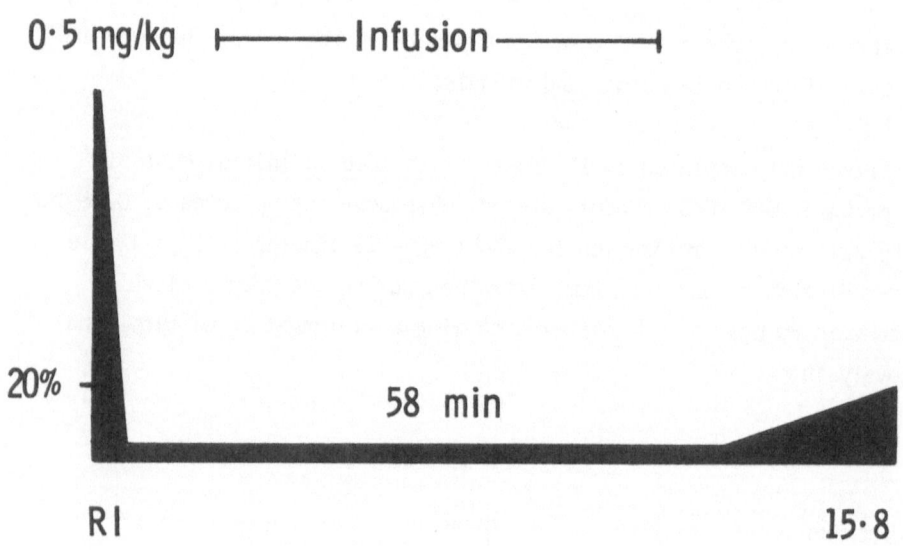

Fig. 5

3. Dr. Hollway and I are at present determining whether a log dose/ duration plot will enable us to predict a suitable large initial bolus to produce relaxation for a given duration. Fig. 6 represents typical durations of block and recovery indexes following the administration of 0.15 mg/Kg and 0.2 mg/Kg.

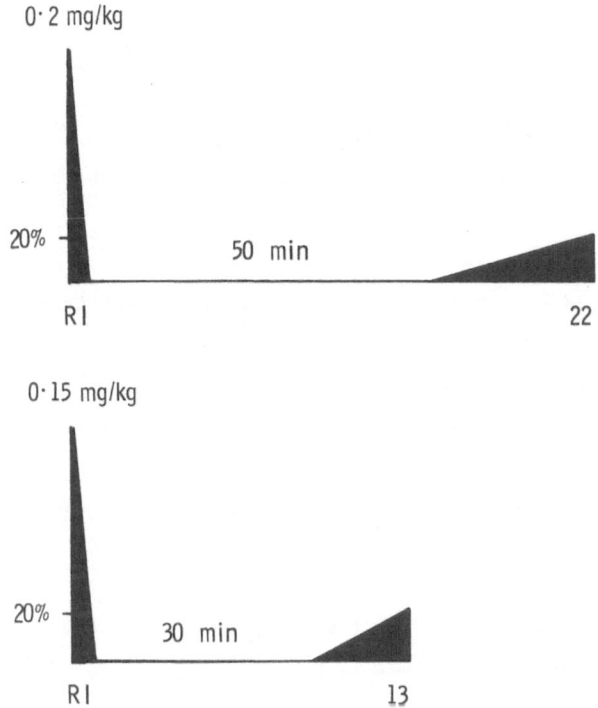

0·2 mg/kg

20%

50 min

R I

22

0·15 mg/kg

20%

30 min

R I

13

Fig. 6

This technique has the advantage of producing relaxation of a
duration longer than with tubocurarine but without its side effects.
However, a larger recovery index occurs when higher doses are
administered.

The important kinetic parameters of ORG NC45 in a clinically useful dose
for an operation lasting about 1 hour, or 0.15 mg/Kg have been provided
by Dr. Bencini.   He has shown an $\tilde{\alpha}$ half-life of 2.0 min. , a β half-
life of 12.17 and a δ half-life of 112.3 min.   These figures are in
keeping with the clinical duration of action observed and explain why
some prolongation of the recovery index is found with higher dose levels.

A new generation of neuromuscular blocking agents are about to be introduced into anaesthesia. Sensibly used they will meet at least two of Saverese and Kitz's criteria and because of their specificity and lack of cumulative effect they should be safer and more convenient to use.

REFERENCES

1. Goat V.A. and Feldman S.A. (1972) The effect of non-depolarizing muscle relaxants on the cholinergic mechanism of the isolated rabbit heart. Anaesthesia 27.149.

2. Parmentier P. and Dagrelie P. (1979) Dose related tachycardia produced by pancuronium during balanced anaesthesia with and without droperidol. Brit. J. Anaesth. 51.157.

3. Bonta I.L., Goarissen E.M. and Derkx F.N. (1968) Pharmacological interactions between pancuronium bromide and anaesthetics. Eur. J. Pharmacol. 4.83.

4. Ivankovitch A.D. et al (1975) The effect of pancuronium on myocardial contraction and catecholamine metabolism. J. Pharm. Pharmacol. 27.837.

5. Conway C.M., Salt P.J. and Barnes P.K. (1979) Inhibition of neuronal uptake of noradrenaline by pancuronium in the isolated perfused rat heart. Brit. J. Anesth. 51.66.

6. Saverese J.J. and Kitz R.J. (1975) Editorial View. Does clinical anaesthesia need new neuromuscular blocking agents. Anesthesiol. 42.236.

7. Feldman S.A. (1973) In Muscle relaxants. Publ. W.B. Saunders (Lond) p. 158.

8. Hughes R. and Chapple D.J. (1980) Experimental studies with atracurium, a new neuromuscular blocking agent. Brit. J. Anesth. 52.238.

9. Hunt T.M., Hughes R. and Payne J.P. (1980) Preliminary studies with atracurium in anesthetised man. Brit. J. Anaesth. 52.238.

10. Savage D.S. (1980) The emergence of Org NC45, from the pancuronium series. Brit. J. Anaesth. 52. suppl. 1.35.

11. Agoston S. et al (1980) The neuromuscular blocking action of Org NC45 a new pancuronium derivative, in anaesthetised patients. A pilot study. Brit. J. Anaesth. 52. Suppl. 1. 53.5.

12. Marshall I.G. et al (1980) Pharmacology of Org NC45 compared with other non-depolarizing neuromuscular blocking drugs. Brit. J. Anaesth. 52. Suppl. 1. 115.

13. Krieg N. et al (1980) Relative potency of Org NC45, pancuronium, alcuronium and tubocurarine in anaesthetised man. Brit. J. Anaesth. 52.738.

14. Agoston S. (1981) Personal communication.

15. Barnes P.K. (1981) Comparison of the effect of Org NC45 and pancuronium on pulse and blood pressure in anaesthetised man. Presented to Anaesthetic Research Soc. May 1981.

16. Harrison P. and Feldman S.A. (1981) Intubating conditions with Orq NC45 to be published in Anaesthesia.

BASIC PHARMACOLOGY AND POSSIBLE THERAPEUTIC APPLICATIONS OF
4-AMINOPYRIDINE

S. AGOSTON

During the past few years much experimental work has been
done in order to clarify the pharmacological profile and
define the clinical usefulness of a relatively old, but
little known, substance, 4-aminopyridine (4-AP). This
compound was developed more than 20 years ago in the U.S.A.
and is used as a bird "repellant". Birds, acutely poisoned,
become disoriented and emit a distress cry which is known as
a signal by other members of the flock to avoid undesirable
places (1).

During the last decades there have been several reports
of the facilitatory actions of the 2-, 3-, and 4-aminopyridines
on transmission at various synapses in both vertebrates and
intervertebrates (2,3,4). More recently, Bulgarian anaesthetists
have described (5) the use of 4-aminopyridine hydrochloride
(Pymadine[R]) as an anticurare agent in anaesthetic practice.
For about ten years 4-AP has been used in Bulgaria as the main
anticurare agent in daily clinical practice.

The topics to be discussed in this lecture will, therefore,
include the basic pharmacology of 4-aminopyridine, including
its mechanism of action, effects at the neuromuscular junction
and skeletal muscle, and in the central nervous system. Its
potential clinical usefulness and toxic effects will be
mentioned as well.

4-Aminopyridine is a lipid soluble quaternary ammonium
compound with various electrophysiologic effects on excitable
membranes. At membrane level the main action of 4-AP is to
decrease membrane potassium conductance. Although highly
ionized at body pH, 4-AP readily penetrates the blood brain
barrier as evidenced by its central stimulant action.

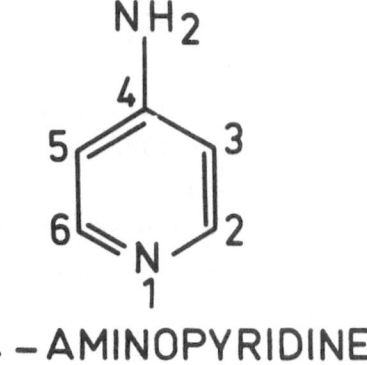

4 – AMINOPYRIDINE

Figure 1. Structural formula 4-aminopyridine.

Before discussing the mechanism of action of this compound, let us review briefly the main factors involved in the transmission processes at the neuromuscular junction and in the contraction of skeletal muscle.

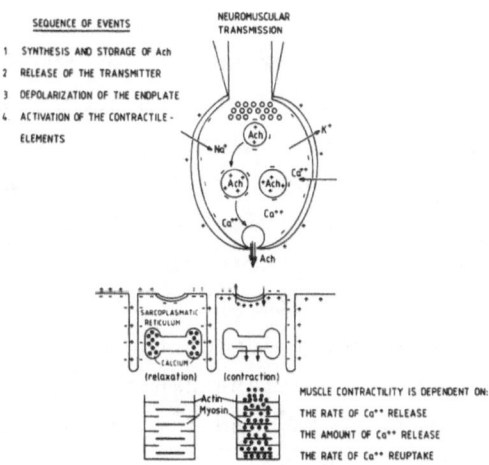

Figure 2. Neuromuscular transmission and muscle contraction.

General

The train of events in neuromuscular transmission starts with the synthesis and storage of acetylcholine (Ach) in the motor nerve terminals. When liberated from this store by the nerve impulse, Ach diffuses across the synaptic cleft and reacts with the receptor molecules at the motor end plate. The formation of this transmitter receptor complex brings about an increased cation permeability of the cell, which leads to a local reduction in membrane potential at the end plate. When this reduction of the end plate potential reaches a critical level, a conducted action potential is initiated in the adjacent muscle fiber membrane, and this action potential causes activation of the contractile elements in the muscle.

Release of the transmitter

Although the dispute about the mechanism of transmitter release is by no means settled as yet - a widely accepted hypothesis holds that acetylcholine is held within the presynaptic vesicles.

The release mechanism involves temporary fusion of the vesicular membrane with the membrane of the nerve terminal, the contents being expelled by exocytosis. Both the outer surface of the synaptic vesicles and the inner surface of the motor nerve terminal are negatively charged. It has been suggested that the two positive charges on a calcium ion serve to neutralize these fixed negative membrane charges, thereby enabling the vesicles to come into contact with the release sites.

Calcium ions play a very important linking role, not only in the release of acetylcholine at the motor nerve ending, but also in the contractile mechanism of the muscle.

Due to the increase in membrane permeability, during the nerve action potential, to Na^+ and K^+, there is a net movement of these cations through the membrane in accordance with their concentration gradients. Most of the current is carried by Na^+ and K^+ ions, moving in opposite directions, but the membrane becomes permeable also to calcium. The entry of calcium occurs immediately after the action potential when the increase in

permeability is still present and the electrical gradient is
favourable. Therefore small changes in the amplitude or in
duration of the action potential will in turn determine the
size and duration of the ionic fluxes - also the inward flux
of calcium ions which activate the release mechanism. It has
been shown (6) that the amount of transmitter released is a
linear function of the inward calcium current.

Excitation - contraction coupling

Acetylcholine released from the nerve endings diffuses across
the synaptic cleft and combines with specific macro-molecules,
called cholinoceptors located on the exterior face of the post-
junctional motor end plate. The result of the acetylcholine/
receptor interaction is depolarization of the end plate. If the
end plate is sufficiently depolarized, the end plate potential
will trigger off an action potential of the muscle which will
ultimately result in the activation of the contractile elements
of the muscle. The chain of events that couple the depolarization
of the muscle cell membrane to activation of the contractile
mechanism is called excitation - contraction coupling.

Muscle contraction

The progress of contraction is a consequence of the formation
of "cross-bridges" between the contractile proteins myosin (thick
filaments) and actin (thin filaments). The thin filaments are
composed mainly of the protein actin - but with a complex of
two other proteins, troponin and tropomyosin, closely associated
with it. At rest (when the amount of free calcium in the sarco-
plasm is low) the troponin-tropomyosin complex inhibits cross-
bridge formation between actin and myosin, so that relaxation
is actively maintained. However, following sufficient depolarization of the end plate the electrical change in the adjacent
muscle cell membrane is conducted into the interior of the
muscle fiber. This electrical change causes the release of
calcium which is at rest stored in the sarcoplasmatic reticulum.
When sufficient calcium is released from the sarcoplasmatic
reticulum, the "blockade" of the cross-bridge formation will

be temporarily lifted since calcium will bind to troponin-
tropomyosin, making actin free for interaction with myosin,
the result of which is the contraction of the muscle. Restoration
of the relaxed state requires that calcium be removed from the
troponin-tropomyosin complex which can then re-exert its inhibitory
actions on cross-bridge formation.

Drugs may increase or decrease the contractions of the striated
muscle by affecting one or more of the processes in the excitation-contraction coupling sequence. The altered contractility
is usually due to a change in:
- the rate of Ca^{++} release
- the amount of Ca^{++} released or
- the rate of Ca^{++} reuptake
by the sarcoplasmatic reticulum.

Mechanism of action of 4-aminopyridine

With the aforementioned in mind, it is very easy to understand
the mechanism of action of 4-AP. Its main effect at the motor
nerve terminal is to decrease membrane potassium conductance.
As an outward potassium current is essential for the repolarization phase of an action potential, such an inhibitory action
of 4-AP results in slowing of the action potential during its
repolarization phase. The prolongation of the duration of the
nerve action potential results in a greater influx of calcium
into the nerve terminal and thus increased release of acetylcholine (7).

In the skeletal muscle 4-AP by direct action, makes more
calcium available for the excitation-contraction coupling, which
ultimately will result in increase of the muscle contractility.
Although 4-AP is known to prolong the duration of the action
potentials of the muscle fibres it is more likely that its
positive inotrope effects on the muscle are due to its direct
action on the membrane calcium channels at the sarcoplasmatic
reticulum facilitating the efflux of calcium ions into sarcoplasmatic reticulum (8).

There is also animal experimental and clinical evidence
indicating some analeptic actions of 4-AP. The central actions

are thought to be mediated by a similar pre-synaptic mechanism
to that seen in the periphery, and are not necessarily restricted
to effects upon any particular type of synapse or transmitter;
although it is probable that central cholinoceptive sites are
most sensitive to the actions of this compound. However, a more
recent report (9) suggests that CNS stimulating effects of 4-AP
might be due to the blockade of purines (adenosine) at the
purinergic receptors.

Clinically useful effects of 4-aminopyridine

4-AP exerts therefore clinically useful facilitatory effects
at least in three biological systems:
- neuromuscular junction
- skeletal muscle
- CNS.

Neuromuscular junction

At the neuromuscular junction 4-AP increases the release of
acetylcholine. This presynaptic action is helpful in reversing
the neuromuscular effects of certain antibiotics like neomycin
and streptomycin since they act presynaptically by decreasing
acetylcholine release.

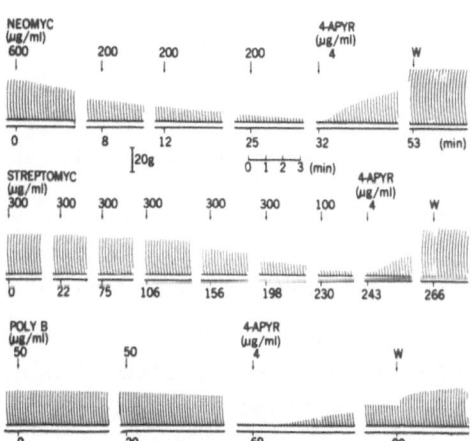

Figure 3.
Burkett
et al.,
1979 (10).

Comparison of the antagonist effect of 4-aminopyridine
(4-APYR) on neuromuscular block induced by neomycin, streptomycin, or polymyxin B. Note that 4-APYR more effectively
antagonized neomycin and streptomycin than polymyxin B.

210

In figure 3 the antagonist effect of 4-AP on neuromuscular
block induced by neomycin, streptomycin and polymixin B is
compared in the rat in vitro (10). Note that 4-AP more effectively
reversed neomycin and streptomycin than polymixin B which suggests
that the affinity of these polypeptide antibiotics for sites of
acetylcholine release may be greater than that of aminoglycosides.
Increased amounts of acetylcholine at the neuromuscular junction,
no matter whether due to increased release or by accumulation
due to inhibited breakdown, will antagonize partial neuromuscular
blockade due to non-depolarizing muscle relaxants.

Such an effect is shown in figure 4.

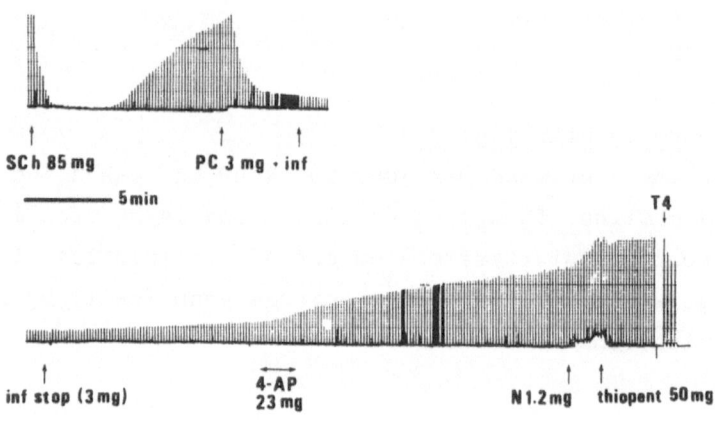

Figure 4. Reversal of pancuronium (Pc) induced neuromuscular blockade by 4-aminopyridine and
neostigmine (from Dr Y. Sohn, 1981)(11).

This is a record of a patient who underwent a gynaecological
operation under neurolept anaesthesia. After full recovery of
the suxamethonium induced paralysis a dose of pancuronium
30 µg/kg was administered, followed by a continuous infusion
of pancuronium to produce and maintain a constant 90 percent
depression of twitch tension. After the peritoneal closure, the
infusion was stopped to allow partial spontaneous recovery.

When the twitch tension recovered to 20% of control, 230 µg/kg
4-AP was injected in a 2 min period. As a result the recovery
rate increased; however, there was less than 80% recovery by
15 min, and therefore, neostigmine 12 µg/kg was given together
with atropine which resulted in a prompt and complete restoration
of the neuromuscular transmission within a few minutes after
the injection. This patient had muscular movements probably due
to awakening as a result of the analeptic action of 4-AP, which
stopped after thiopental. In this case in the presence of a full
antagonizing dose of 4-AP the recovery to 80% lasted 15 mins.
Under similar conditions, without an antagonist, the recovery
of pancuronium would have lasted at least 80-100 mins.

In order to speed up recovery maybe higher doses of 4-AP should
be used. However, 300 µg/kg is the highest safe dose - higher
doses were shown to stimulate the central nervous system (12)
and cause post-operative restlessness and confusion.

4-AP increases acetylcholine release - anticholinesterases
inhibit its breakdown - so it can be expected that when administered together they will mutually potentiate the antagonistic effect
of each other. In other words, the effects of combinations of
4-AP with neostigmine or pyridostigmine can be expected to be
greater than would have been predicted from the sum of the effects
of the individual compounds. Consequently the doses of one or both
drugs in such a combination can be diminished without loss in
antagonistic activity, with considerably lessened risks of side
effects.

The synergism between 4-AP and the cholinesterase inhibitors
was demonstrated in a clinical study (13) in which a steady
state neuromuscular blockade of 90% was produced and maintained
by the infusion of pancuronium bromide. Unlike the previous
study, in this investigation spontaneous recovery was not allowed;
the antagonist was given during the continuous infusion of the
relaxant. Under these experimental conditions the dose of
350 µg/kg 4-AP when given alone appeared to be ineffective.
A dose of 500 µg/kg produced 24% antagonism only, however, with
central nervous system excitation at the same time. When, however,
this by itself ineffective dose of 350 µg/kg 4-AP was combined

212

with neostigmine or pyridostigmine, tremendous potentiation of
their effects could be demonstrated.

In combination with the above dose of 4-AP the doses of
neostigmine and pyridostigmine producing 50% antagonism could
be reduced by 70 and 80% respectively.

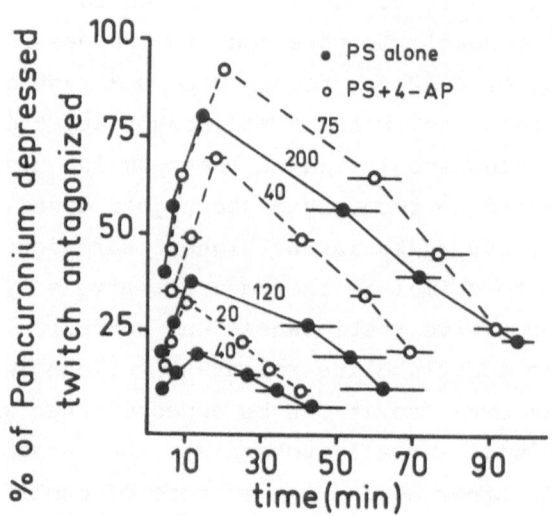

Figure 5. Plot of time and percentage of pancuronium
induced depression of twitch tension antagonized.
The numbers present the doses of pyridostigmine
in µg/kg. The dose of 4-AP used was 350 µg/kg.
Three patients were studied at each dose.
(From: R.D. Miller et al., 1979) (13).

Skeletal muscle

Besides its facilitatory effects at the neuromuscular junction
4-AP exerts also a direct effect on the skeletal muscle increasing
its contractility, which is shown in figure 6. This figure shows
in the cat the antagonistic effects of 4-AP of the muscle
paralysis produced by 2 mg/kg dantrolene sodium. Note that the
muscle action potentials simultaneously recorded remained
unchanged, even after the development of the maximum twitch
height depression due to dantrolene. This supports the earlier

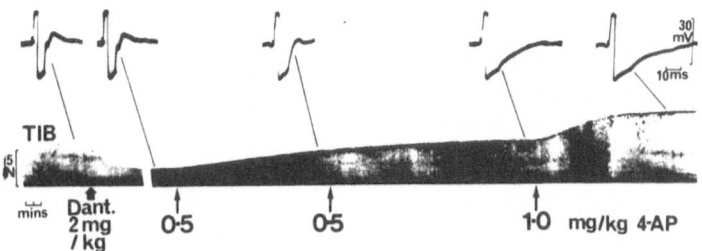

Figure 6. Maximal twitches and gross muscle action
potentials of a tibialis anterior muscle
evoked by stimulation of the motor nerve.
At DANT, dantrolene sodium, and at the
remaining arrows 4-AP were injected intravenously.
(From: W.C. Bowman) (14).

findings that dantrolene exerts its effect beyond the end plate
and does not interfere with neuromuscular transmission. In
contrast, the administration of incremental doses of 4-AP reversed
the twitch height depression and prolonged the duration of the
muscle action potentials at the same time in a dose-dependent
fashion. This is in full agreement with the known facts regarding
the mechanism of action of 4-AP. Since dantrolene is known to act
by inhibition of the release of calcium from the sarcoplasmatic
reticulum (15), the reversal of dantrolene induced muscle
relaxation by 4-AP indicates that 4-AP also facilitates the
exitation - contraction coupling processes in skeletal muscle (8).
This effect of 4-AP is entirely different from and complementary
to its pre-synaptic actions by which the curare-like agents are
antagonized.

Central nervous system (CNS)

The next biological system where 4-AP may have clinically
useful facilitatory actions is the brain. The analeptic effects
of 4-AP were already suggested by the Bulgarian clinical
investigators (5). We studied (16) the effects of 4-AP on the
CNS in cats by measuring the quantified phrenic nerve activity
as an indication of the central respiratory drive. In this study

4-AP 1 mg/kg increased spontaneous phrenic nerve activity by
approximately 30% (figure 7). This effect could be abolished
within 2-3 mins by high doses of atropine (1 mg/kg) indicating
the involvement of central cholinergic mechanisms.

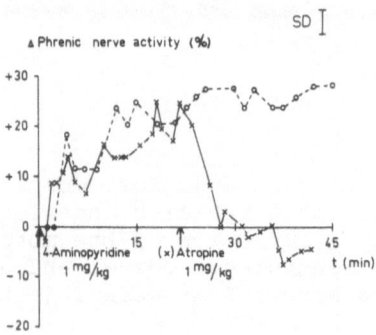

Fig.7. Effect of administration of 4-aminopyridine (1 mg/kg) on
the phrenic nerve activity. With (×   —×) and without (O——O)
subsequent administration of atropine (1 mg/kg). The increase in
activity after 4-aminopyridine was completely abolished within
2−3 min by atropine. The results of two different animals are plotted
in this figure

(From: Folgering et al., 1979) (16).

In a clinical study designed to elucidate the central nervous
system stimulation by 4-AP, Sia (17) and other members of our
Research Group in Groningen have demonstrated the ability of
4-AP to reverse opiate-induced respiratory depression in
patients. Their findings are summarized in figure 8.

The PCO_2, PO_2, tidal volumes, respiratory rate and the
occlusion pressure were measured before, four mins after the
administration of either morphine or fentanyl, and 2 and 4 mins
following the administration of 4-AP. All patients who received
one of these opiates showed apnoea followed by a slow and shallow
respiratory pattern. After the administration of 4-AP there was
a statistically significant improvement in all parameters. The
tidal volume was doubled and approached the control values after
the administration of 300 µg/kg 4-AP. Also significant improvement
was seen in the occlusion pressure which was found, also by other
investigators, to be a reliable index of respiratory drive in

anaesthetized patients.

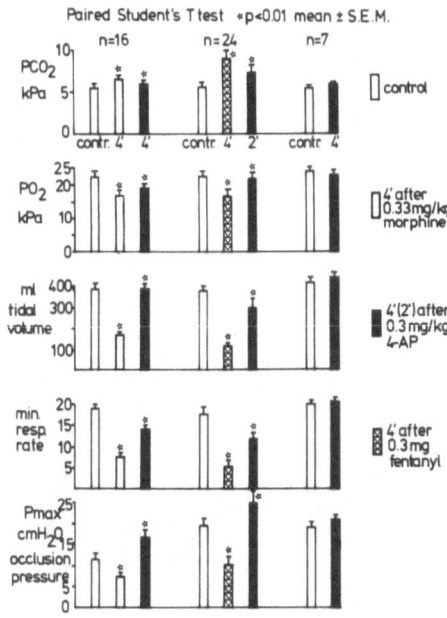

Figure 8. Effects of 4-AP upon morphine or fentanyl
depressed respiration. (From R. Sia, 1980).

In another investigation in human volunteers (18) we have
shown that 4-AP (300 µg/kg) increases the rate of recovery of
subjects from diazepam/ketamine anaesthesia. The volunteers
were given 2 mg/kg ketamine preceded by diazepam 0.2 mg/kg
intravenously. After the ketamine bolus injection each volunteer
received ketamine 1 mg/kg/h by intravenous infusion for one
hour. Ten mins after stopping the infusion the volunteers were
tested and then either 4-AP or the same volume of saline was
administered. Each volunteer served as his own control,
receiving 4-AP or saline on two different occasions. The results
on these experiments have shown a drastic shortening of the
mean times required for the successful completion of tests
employed, following the administration of saline or 4-AP
respectively (figure 9).

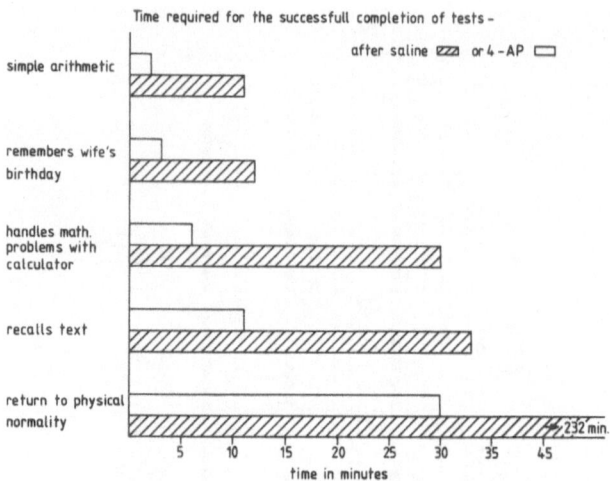

Figure 9. (From Agoston et al., 1980) (18).

Summary and conclusions

Many of the various actions of 4-AP could be useful in
daily anaesthetic practice. Its presynaptic effects, resulting
in an enormous increase in acetylcholine release, are successfully used to antagonize partial neuromuscular blockade not only
due to antibiotics and neuromuscular blocking agents, but also
in cases of impaired neuromuscular transmission due to Botulinus
intoxication (12). Encouraging reports appeared recently on
the use of 4-AP in patients with Eaton-Lambert syndrome (19)
and Myasthenia gravis (20). The potentiation of the effects of
neostigmine and pyridostigmine by 4-AP makes it possible to use
smaller than usual doses of these compounds when combined with
4-AP. Combinations of relatively small doses of 4-AP and anticholinesterases may elevate acetylcholine concentration at the
neuromuscular junction to the same or higher levels than larger
doses of the individual compounds. In addition, the use of small
doses in combination most probably will attenuate or eliminate
the disadvantages that these drugs have when given individually.

The analeptic effect of 4-AP - reversing opiate induced

respiratory depression - would by no means justify its use as an opiate antagonist, but this effect together with its anti-curare actions could be beneficial at the end of the surgery.

One of the major shortcomings of 4-AP is its narrow therapeutic index; doses higher than 800 µg/kg are likely to produce toxic effects (21) including restlessness, confusion, nausea, weakness and generalized tonic-clonic seizures. High doses of diazepam up to 80 mg i.v. (12) successfully alleviated these effects.

In conclusion, I would like to stress that actions at various sites on different biological systems of any compound, may complicate and limit its clinical use by increased risks of dangerous side effects and interactions. However, the properties of 4-AP including antagonism of non-depolarizing block by increasing presynaptic acetylcholine release and the contractility of skeletal muscle, in addition to the reversal of central nervous system depression due to certain anaesthetics and opiates - are potentially promising features, especially for anaesthesiologists, and warrant, therefore, further extensive studies in animal and man.

REFERENCES

1. Schafer EW et al. 1973. A summary of acute toxicity of 4-aminopyridine to birds and mammals. Tox Appl Pharm 20, 532-538.
2. Fastier FN and McDowal NA. 1958. A comparison of the pharmacological properties of the three isomeric amino-pyridines. Austral J exp Biol 36, 365-372.
3. Lemeignan M et al. 1969. Etude de l'action d'un convulsivant spécial (la 4-aminopyridine) sur les nerfs de vertebrés. CR Soc Biol (Paris) 163, 359-365.
4. Molgo J et al. 1975. Modifications de la liberation du transmitteur à la jonction neuromusculaire de grenouille sous l'action de l'amino-4-pyridine. CD Acad Sci (Paris) D. 281, 1637-1639.
5. Paskov DS et al. 1973. New anticurare and analeptic drug Pimadin (4-aminopyridine hydrochloride) and its use in anaesthesia (in Russian). Eksper Khir Anesthesiol 18, 48-52.
6. Llinás R. 1977. Calcium and transmitter release in squid synapse. In: Cowan WM and Ferrendelli JA (eds). Society for Neuroscience Symposia, vol. II. Approaches to the cell biology of neurons. Bethesda, Maryland, Society for Neuro-science, pp. 139-160.
7. Lundh H et al. 1977. Antagonism of the paralysis produced by botulinum toxin in the rat. The effects of tetra-aethyl-

ammonium, guanidine and 4-aminopyridine. J Neurol Sci 32, 29-43.

8. Agoston S et al. 1981. Direct action of 4-aminopyridine on the contractility of a fast contracting muscle in the cat. Clin Exp Pharm & Physiol (in press).

9. Perkins MN and Stone TW. 1980. 4-aminopyridine blockade of neuronal depressant responses to adenosine triphosphate. Br J Pharmac 70, 425-428.

10. Burkett L et al. 1979. Mutual potentiation of the neuro-muscular effects of antibiotics and relaxants. Anesth Analg 58, 107-115.

11. Ball AP et al. 1979. Human botulism caused by Clostridium botulinum, type E: The Birmingham outbreak. Quaterly J Med 191, 473-491.

12. Sohn YJ. 1981. Personal communication.

13. Miller RD et al. 1979. 4-aminopyridine potentiates neostigmine and pyridostigmine in man. Anesthesiology 50, 416-420.

14. Bowman WC. 1979. Personal communication.

15. Ellis KO and Carpenter JF. 1972. Studies on the mechanism of action of dantrolene sodium. A skeletal muscle relaxant. Naunyn-Schmiedeberg's Arch exp Path Pharmac 275, 83-87.

16. Folgering H et al. 1979. Stimulation of phrenic nerve activity by an acetylcholine releasing drug: 4-aminopyridine. Pflügers Archiv 379, 181-185.

17. Sia RL and Zandstra DF. 1981. 4-aminopyridine reversal of morphine-induced respiratory depression in human. Br J Anaesth (in press).

18. Agoston S et al. 1980. Antagonism of ketamine-diazepam anaesthesia by 4-aminopyridine in human volunteers. Br J Anaesth 52, 367-370.

19. Agoston S et al. 1978. Effects of 4-aminopyridine in Eaton-Lambert syndrome. Br J Anaesth 50, 383-385.

20. Kim YJ et al. 1980. Facilitatory effects of 4-aminopyridine on neuromuscular transmission in disease states. Muscle & Nerve 3, 112-119.

21. Spijker DA et al. 1980. Poisoning with 4-aminopyridine: A report of three cases. Clin Toxicol 16, 487-497.

THE EPIDURAL USE OF NARCOTIC ANALGESICS

J.T. Davidson

The immense potential benefits which the juice of the unripe
poppy seed could bestow on suffering mankind have not been fully
realized because of the perils of the side effects. Time and
time again new surrogates and derivatives have been presented
which supposedly have morphine-like properties without addiction
or central depression. Two examples are heroin introduced as
non-addictive about 1890, and pethidine 50 years later with a
similar claim. It seemed that the linkage between therapeutic
value and risk was inexorable and inextricable.

Recently a new attempt has been made in pain control using
opiates by the intrathecal(1) and epidural (2) routes. In
this presentation the theoretical background willbe reviewed and
an assessment will be made of the applicability, efficacy and
safety in acutely painful states.

Opiate Receptors and Endorphins

The spinal (i.e. epidural and intrathecal) use of opiates was
prompted by important developments in our conception of the
site of action of the narcotic analgesics,particularly by the
identification of specific opiate binding sites or recetors
(3,4,5). The presence of these receptors has been suspected
for many years because of the basic similarity in molecular
structure found in the thousands of opiates. These exist in
two optical isomers - mirror image molecules identical in
chemical composition and molecular weight - but only the
levorotary isomer possesses thecharacteristics of the narcotic
analgesics. Furthermore three classes of opiates are
recognized; agonists, antagonists and mixed agonists -
antagonists. Pharmacological differences between these classes
is very pronounced while the molecular modifications necessary
to change from agonist to antagonist are slight. All this
suggests that the opiate seeks out selective receptor sites
with the antagonist competing with the agonist for access to

the receptor molecule. A conceptual problem arose when in vitro experiments appeared to demonstrate that agonists and antagonists bind with equal affinity to the receptors - a fact which conflicts with the clinical finding that antagonists such as naloxone are much more potent than narcotics. This apparent contradiction was resolved when Snyder (6) demonstrated that sodium in concentrations normally found in the body alters the receptors in such a way that the affinity of the antagonists is increased and of the agonist decreased.

The strong affinity binding sites are unequally distributed in the central nervous system. Dense concentrations have been demonstrated in the peri-aqueductal grey, the hypothalamus the medial thalamus and the substantia gelatinosa of the cord (7,8).

The presence of highly specific opiate receptors in the central nervous system was suggestive of an interation with endogenous opiates. This line of reasoning was authenticated by the isolation from brain of two pentapeptides with analgesic actively (9). These were named enkephalins ("in the head") and their distribution corresponds to that of the opiate receptors. Other endorphins (endogenous morphine) have been subsequently isolated and purified. These include beta-endorphin from the pituitary (10) which is a cleavage product of the precursor peptide for ACTH, and may have a role in the regulation of pituitary function. The physiological role of the enkephalin/endorphin system is still largely speculative. Electrical stimulation or the peri-aqueductal grey has been shown to generate naloxone reversible analgesia. "This stimulation analgesia" is accompanied by a release of endorphins into the cerebrospinal fluid (11,12). These findings give support for the supposition that modulation of pain perception is a function of the system and may provide a physiological basis for differences in perception of painful stimuli. Petrie (13) demonstrated that each individual has a characteristic perceptual reactance to pain with a tendancy to enlarge (augmentation) or diminish (reduction) what is being experienced. Knorring et al (14) found that augmenters have significantly lower levels of endorphins

in their cerebrospinal fluid than reducers. This observed
association between endorphin level and pain sensitivity
strengthens the concept that endorphins function as endogenous
antinociceptors.

It is unlikely, however, that pain threshold is a fixed entity.
there is evidence that sensitivity to aversive stimuli may
decrease during some forms of stress. Thus Gintzler demonstrated
(15) that during pregnancy there is a gradual rise in the
pain threshold of rats which reaches its peak close to
parturition. The fact that this rise was prevented by a
narcotic antagonist strongly suggests that the relative
insensitivity to pain noted could be ascribed to the activation
of the endorphin system.

Characteristics and Mechanism of Spinal Narcotic Block
It is firmly established that the nociceptive threshold is
elevated leading to prolonged analgesia both in laboratory
animals (16) and in man (1,2,17) even when the blood levels
are below those which support analgesia (18,26). This
strongly suggests a local action on the spinal cord and bears
on the long standing controversy as to whether opiate analgesia
is mediated only in the brain, or acts also on the cord.
The observation, many years ago, that in human subjects with
complete spinal cord transection systemic morphine depresses
nocioceptive flexor withdrawal reflexes infered that the site
was not entirely supraspinal. This view is now corroborated.

High levels of opiate binding have been demonstrated in the
substantia gelatinosa of the cord. Here the small diameter
primary afferents (C fibres) synapse with the second order
neurones, and destruction of this primary afferent imput by
rhizory leads to a significant fall in opiate binding in the
region. The opiate alters favourably the configuration of
the endogeous inhibitory pain system perhaps by blocking the
segmental secretion of a putative transmitter, substance P (19),
or by releasing encephalins (20), or by restoring neural
transmitters depleted by stress or chronic pain (21).

Whatever the mechanism the rostral transmission of nociceptive
information is antagonised. It is significant that there is a dense
concentration of opiate receptors in association with the
paleospinothalamic tract which conducts the poorly localized
deep burning pain recognized to be much more amenable to morphine,
than the sharp localized pain transmitted through the more laterally
placed neospinothalamic pathway.

Characteristically pain relief following narcotics is not
accompanied by perceptible loss of sensory, motor, propriceptive
or autonomic function. This is in keeping with the concept that
opiates administered by the intrathecal or epidural routes act on a
single receptor system. In contrast to local anaethesia there is no
depolarization of the neurone membrane.

The latency and duration of action of the different narcotics given
by the spinal route depend on the physico - chemical characteristics.
Thus epidural morphine with its large, highly ionized molecule, low
lipoid solubility and low protein binding has a long latency of
onset (about 20 minutes) and a prolonged action (8-10 hours)
relative to equipotent dose of fentanyl. Adrenaline 1/200,000 has
not been found to prolong epidural narcotic analgesia (22).

Spinal tolerance has been reported after repeated epidural
administration of narcotics. Thus the drug may be almost non-active
after the 5th day (23). However there are conflicting reports on
this phenomenon.

The existence of a sensory segmental level is much less clear cut
than obtained after local analgesics. However Bromage and
colleagues (24) were able to detect in volunteers a level using pin-
scratch and cold stimuli. Asari et al (25) established the
clinical relevance of the segmental effect of epidural morphine in
the post-operative stage. They demonstrated that morphine injected
at tenth to eleventh thoracic interspace was more effective for pain
relief after upper abdominal surgery, than a similar dose injected
between the fifth lumbar and first sacral vertebrae.

Weddel et al (26) recently attempted to correlate serum levels of morphine, after epidural administration, with post-surgical pain relief. They found that neither the onset, the duration nor the intensity of analgesia correlated well with blood levels after epidural narcotic. This finding gives strong support to the concept of a direct spinal action.

Sexual affects may be important in patients receiving prolonged therapy. Potency is apparently unimpaired although an inability to ejaculate has been reported.(27).

Clinical Application

Epidural narcotics have been used in a wide range of cases in order to define its sphere of usefulness in acute pain. The table summarizes our experiences with 2-4mgs. morphine without preservatives or stabilizers and used within one month of preparation. The result is defined as "good" if at least 80% of the patients being treated did not require futher analgesia for a minimum of 5 hours, and"fair" if between 50-80% were in that category. The result is "poor" if less than 50% obtained 5 hour relief.

Experience with Epidural Morphine

INDICATION	NO OF PATIENTS	RESULT
Post operative	210	Good
Labour pain		
1) Full term	18	Poor
2) 2nd trimester induced abortion	16	Good
Fractured Ribs	7	Good
Renal stones	7	Good
Malignancy	53	Good
Low back pain	31	Fair
Ischemic pain	6	Good
Causalgia	5	Poor
Phantom pain	2	Good

Total: 355

Post-operative pain

Epidural morphine has its widest application in the field of
post-operative pain. In contrast to the state after systemic
narcotics, the patient is alert and analgesia is intense not only
at rest but also during movement. Thus deep breathing and
coughing after abdominal and thoracic surgery as well as early
ambulation, cause no distress. It has also been shown to be
effective for the very severe pain following orthopaedic
proceedures such as arthrotomy, allowing the early commencement
of pain-free rehabilitation therapy (28).

Bromage and his colleagues (22) measures forced expiratory volume
in one second (FEV_1) as an index of respiratory function after
upper abdominal and thoracic surgery. They found that following
epidural morphine, FEV_1 improved from 37% of pre-operative values
to 67%. The corresponding rise after intravenous morphine was to
44%. Torda et al (27) determined the CO_2 response curve in
healthy volunteers after the epidural administration of 3-4mgs.
morphine and found no statistically significant depression over a
3 hour period. This is in keeping with the finding of Chayen et al(23)
that epidural morphine after surgery or trauma was not associated with
ventilatory problems, and that, specifically, tidal volume was
within normal range. While respiratory depression does not therefore
appear to be a feature of epidural narcotics within the usual dose
range, inadvert subarachnoid injection through a misplaced
catheter carries this hazard (29).

We conducted a double blind study on post-operative pain control
in 65 patients after Caesarian section, 40 of whom received 4mgs.
morphine administered through an epidural catheter and 25 acted as
controls receiving no epidural analgesia. 67% of the experimental
group required no supplementart narcotics for 8-12 hours, and
22% remained pain free for the 24 hours of observation. Most of
the controls required systemic narcotics within 4 hours (30).

Labour pain

We found that the pain relief resulting from epidural morphine in doses up to 4mgs. was decidely poor (17). Confirmation of this finding has come from other centres (31,32). This is explained by the fact that epidural narcotic acts on a single receptor system (small c fibres) leaving motor and sympathetic conduction intact. On the other hand the technique was much more successful in abolishing labour pain in second-trimester induced abortion (33).

Fractured ribs

Both the post traumatic chest pain and the PaO_2 were dramatically improved. Ventilation in flail chest became slower and more efficient so that the need for mechanical ventilation was obviated (17).

Summary

In acutely painful situations epidural morphine has its widest application in the field of post-operative pain relief, which is achieved by blockade of transmission along a single receptor system subserving pain. Thus, in contrast to conduction block with local anaethetics there is no loss of touch, propriocetion or motor block, and analgesia is achieved without a "wooden" sensation. Further more there is no chemical sympathectomy to mitigate against early ambulation. The total dose of morphine administrated over a 24 hour period represents an 80-90% reduction as compared to accepted routines of intramuscular morphine used after surgery. Hence the patient is more alert and able to co-operate in rehabilitation programs at an early stage.
There is also an important field of usefulness in the management of fractured ribs and renal stones. Thus the use of epidural narcotics is a significant therapeutic breakthrough in that effective analgesia is achieved without general intoxication. It appears that the iron bond between the analgesic effect of the narcotics and their serious side effects may be loosened.

REFERENCES

1. Wang J.K., Nauss L.A., Thomas J.E., Pain relief by intrathecally applied morphines in humans. Anesthesiology (50): 149-151, 1979.
2. Behar M., Magora F., Olshwang D., Davidson J.T., Epidural morphine in treatment of pain. Lancet (1):527-528, 1979.
3. Pert G.B., Snyder S.H., Opiate receptors: Demonstration in nervous tissue. Science (179): 1011-1014, 1973.
4. Terenius L., Characteristics of the"receptor" for narcotic analgesics in synaptic plasma membrane fraction from rat brain. Acta Pharmacol (33): 377-384, 1973.
5. Simon E.J., Hiller J.M., Edelman I., Stereospecific binding of the potent narcotic analgesic H-Etorphine to rat-brain homogenate. Proc. Natl Acad Sci (USA)(70): 1947-1949, 1973.
6. Snyder S.H. Opiate receptors and internal opiates. Scientific American (236): 44-66, 1977.
7. Kuhar M.J., Pert C.B., Snyder S.H., Regional distribution of opiate receptor binding in monkey and human brain. Nature (245): 447-450, 1973.
8. Pert C.B., Kuhar M.J., Snyder S.H., Opiate Receptor: Autoradiographic localization in rat brain. Proc Natl Acad Sci (USA) (73): 3729-3733, 1976.
9. Hughes J., Smith T.W., Kosterlitz H.W. et al. Identification of two related pentapeptides from the brain with potent opiate agonist activity. Nature (258): 577-579, 1975.
10. Cox B.M., Goldstein A., Li C.H.,Opioid activity of a peptide, beta-endorphin(61-91), derived from beta-lipoprotein. Proc. Natl Acad Sci (USA) (73): 1821-1823, 1973.
11. Mayer D.J., Leibeskind J.C., Pain reduction by focal electrical stimulation of the brain an anatomical and behavioral analysis. Brain Res(68): 73-93, 1974.
12. Akil H., Mayer D.J., Liebeskind J.C., Antagonism of stimulation produced analgesia by naloxone, a narcotic antagonist. Science 961-962, 1976.
13. Petrie E.A., Individuality in pain and suffering. University of Chicago Press, Chicago and London, 1967.
14. Knorring L von, Almay B.G.L., Johansson F., Terenius L., Endorphins in CSF of chronic pain patients in relation to augmentation - reducing response in visual averaged evoked response. Neuropsychobiology (5): 322-326 1979.
15. Gintzler A.R. Endorphin-mediated increases in pain threshold during pregnancy. Science (210): 193-195, 1980.
16. Yaksh T.L., Rudy T.A., Studies of the direct spinal action of narcotics in the production of analgesia in the rat. J. Pharmacol. Exp. Ther.(202): 411-428, 1977.
17. Magora F.,Olshwang D,,Eimerl D., Shorr J., Katzenelson R., Cotev S., Davidson J.T., Observations on extradural morphine analgesia in various pain conditions. Br. J. Anaesth (52), 247-252. 1980.
18. Cousins M.J., Mather L.E., Glynn C.J., Wilson F.R., Graham J.R., Selective spinal analgesia. Lancet (1): 1141-? 1979.
19. Jessel J.M., Iversen S.S., Opiate analgesics inhibit substance P release from rat trigeminal nucleus. Nature (268): 549-551, 1977.
20. Sjölund B., Terenius L., Eriksson M., Increased cerebrospinal fluid levels of endorphins after electro-acupuncture Acta Physiol. Scand. (100):382, 1977.

21. Bergmann F., Altstetter R. Weissman B.A., In vivo interaction of morphine and endogenous opiate-like peptides. Life Sciences (23): 2601-2608, 1978.
22. Bromage P.R., Camporesi E., Chestnut D., Epidural narcotics for post-operative analgesia. Anesth Analg. (59): 473-480, 1980.
23. Chayen M.S., Rudick V., Borvine A., Pain control with epidural injection of morphine. Anesthesiology (53): 338-339, 1980.
24. Bromage P.R., Camporesi E., Leslie J., Epidural narcotics in volunteers: sensitivity to pain and to carbon dioxide. Pain (9): 145-160, 1980.
25. Asari H., Inoue K., Shibata J., Soga T., Segmental effect of morphine injected into the epidural space in man. Anesthesiology (54): 75-77, 1981.
26. Weddel S.J., Ritter R.R., Serum levels following epidural administration of morphine and correlation with relief of postsurgical pain. Anesthesiology (54):210-214, 1981.
27. Torda T.A., Pybus D.A., Liberman H., Clark M., Crawford M., Experimental comparison of extradural and I.M. morphine. Br. J. Anaesth. (52): 939-942, 1980.
28. Ebert J., Varner P.D., The effective use of epidural morphine sulphate for postoperative orthopedic pain. Anesthesiology (53): 257-258, 1980.
29. Sidi A., Davidson J.T., Behar M., Olshwang D., Spinal narcotics and central nervous system depression. Anaesthesia. In Press 1981.
30. Donchin Y., Davidson J.T., Magora F., Epidural morphine for the control of pain after Cesarian section. Israel J. Med Sciences. In press 1981.
31. Huseymeyer R.P., O'Connor M.C., Davenport H.C., Failure of epidural morphine to relieve pain in labour. Anaesthesia (35): 161-163, 1980.
32. Stoelting R.K. Opiate receptors and endorphins: Their role in anesthesiology. Anesth. Analg. (59): 874-880, 1980.
33. Magora F., Donchin Y., Olshwang D., Shenkar Y., Epidural morphine in second trimester induced abortion. Amer J. Obstet. Gynec. (138): 260-263, 1980.

WHAT IS NEW IN LOCAL ANESTHESIA?

D.C. Moore

EQUIPMENT

There has been little or no improvement in the quality of single-use (dis-
posable) equipment, with the exception of the following.

■Needles: The 30-gauge, 1.3 cm single-use needle is superb for making
skin wheals painlessly and locally infiltrating the subcutaneous tissue.
While the insertion of this needle into the dermis is painless, injecting
solutions through it to produce the "orange peel" appearance of the skin
does sting.

During 1980 a 22-gauge, 3.8 cm single-use needle with a short bevel (2mm)
and a security bead became available. This needle is comparable in quality to a similar reusable needle, but its point enters the skin much more
easily. These two needles can be obtained from Becton-Dickinson and
Company, Rutherford, New Jersey 07070 USA, and should be in every single-
use regional block tray.

■Plastic Tubing: In its experimental stages is plastic tubing for intermittent (continuous) injection techniques that contains imbedded wire
to stiffen it so that the tubing can be easily threaded through the
needle and the needle withdrawn over it without displacing the tubing.
This would eliminate the use of a stylet to stiffen such tubing. However,
if such tubing were unintentionally "sheared" off, it is not known whether
the remaining piece would cause tissue damage.

■Filters: Glass particles have been found in the solution contained in
ampules after they were opened. Also, after solutions have been emptied
into plastic cups, plastic particles have been seen floating on the surface of the solution. To avoid injecting such particles, as well as contamination should the syringe disconnect from the plastic tubing when
administering a reinforcing (refill, "top-up") dose in an intermittent-

technique, a filter can be used. Initially the filters contained no locking mechanism. When a locking mechanism was devised, it was put on the wrong side of the filter to prevent contamination during an intermittent technique--that is, it was put on the side which attaches to the syringe. Now a filter is available with a locking mechanism on both sides (Abbott Laboratories). Also, a needle is available with a filter in its hub, which screens out glass and plastic particles when filling a syringe (Jelco).

CARDIOTOXICITY OF LOCAL ANESTHETIC DRUGS

In an editorial, Albright theorized that six "anecdotal" cases of convulsions with cardiac arrest were a result of the myocardial depressant effects of etidocaine (Duranest*) and bupivacaine (Marcaine*), not of "antecedent" hypoxia.[1] His statement that these patients were "under the direct supervision of anesthesiologists" should not be construed to imply that the administration of the regional block and/or the treatment of the resulting complication were correct, or that severe hypoxia and acidosis were not the cause of the cardiac arrest.[2]

■Number of Blocks and Dosage: From 1966 through 1980 bupivacaine has been used by us in 21,352 patients for the following blocks: (1) epidural (lumbar and caudal) 12,091; (2) spinal 221; and (3) peripheral nerve (intercostal nerve 5,527, and others 3,513).

Dosages of bupivacaine range as follows: (1) epidural 100 to 225 mg; (2) spinal, 7.5 to 12 mg; and (3) peripheral nerve--brachial 200 to 300 mg; sciatic, femoral, and lateral femoral with or without obturator 300 to 450 mg; and intercostal nerve 275 to 450 mg. In selected cases as much as 675 mg has been used. Many of these intercostal nerve blocks were done in patients whose ASA physical status was scored as 3, 4, or 5. Furthermore, in such patients there was no evidence of cardiotoxicity from bupivacaine as shown by the electrocardioscope, electrocardiogram, or cardiac output determination.

---

*Registered trademark.

I submit that the cases in which an unintentional intravascular bolus dose of local anesthetic drugs has resulted in systemic toxicity with subsequent convulsions, cardiac arrest, brain damage, and death are not a result primarily of cardiotoxicity of such drugs.

■Systemic Toxic Reactions Progressing to Convulsions: Twenty-six major toxic reactions from bupivacaine have resulted (25 convulsions and one bradycardia). Unintentional intravascular bolus doses ranging from 125 to 175 mg following epidural blocks resulted in 23 of the convulsions. Absorption during intercostal nerve block resulted in two convulsions from 250 and 400 mg with epinephrine and one bradycardia from 400 mg without epinephrine.

No cardiac arrest, brain damage, or other sequelae resulted. WHY? Convulsions from bupivacaine are self-limiting because it is detoxified in the liver within a few minutes, as shown by the rapid fall in plasma levels (Table 1). Furthermore, self-limiting convulsions do not cause cardiac arrest, for example, grand mal seizures of epilepsy do not.[3] Untreated or improperly treated severe hypoxia and acidosis, which occur concomittantly with self-limiting convulsions from all local anesthetic drugs, do cause cardiac arrest. The following blood gas data, previously reported, and those from three other patients, confirm that severe hypoxia and acidosis do accompany convulsions (Table 1).[4]

■Prophylactic Therapy to Avoid Systemic Toxicity: In 1925 and 1926, sodium barbital in paraldehyde was shown to protect rabbits, cats, dogs, and monkeys against convulsions from cocaine.[5,6] Whether this protection was from the barbiturates, the paraldehyde, or both was not determined. These investigators cautioned: "The proof of this must of necessity await its clinical application."[5] Nonetheless, without proof in humans, patients were given barbiturates (secobarbital [Seconal*], amobarbital [Amytal*], phenobarbital [Luminal*], pentobarbital [Nembutal*]) orally or intramuscularly prior to the administration of local anesthetic drugs for such preventive effects. In 1974, diazepam (Valium*) was shown to "prevent" convulsions in monkeys.[7] Since then, at least among most anesthesiologists,

---

*Registered trademark.

Table 1

BLOOD GAS DETERMINATIONS
DURING AND AFTER CONVULSIONS

Con-vul-sions	Time	Bupi. ug/ml	02 liters	pH	PCO2	pO2	HCO3	BE
1	0947		10*					
2	0947+ 30 sec	4.4		6.99	76	87	17.4	-10.2
3	0948							
Ceased	0950							
	1003	3.0		7.16	54	140	18.5	-6.9
	1018	2.2	6**	7.26	42	141	18.4	-5.8

*Bag and mask
**Nasal prongs.

diazepam has usurped the place of the barbiturates.

In 1960, we challenged the prophylactic effects of the barbiturates in protecting the human from convulsions from a proper therapeutic dose of the local anesthetic drugs unintentionally injected as a bolus intravascularly.[8] Likewise, we have challenged the prophylactic effects of diazepam in doing so.[2,9,10] Whether this applies to convulsions from absorption is debatable, because the incidence of such reactions in our experience is a rarity and the data, therefore, are insufficient.

Again, let it be emphasized that if barbiturates and diazepam are administered to humans in doses based on extrapolated animal data for the primary purpose of preventing systemic toxicity from local anesthetic drugs, then the physician doing so is being led into a sense of false security. If these drugs can prevent toxicity in humans, then dosages, method of administration, and time of administration as related to the injection of the local anesthetic drug remain to be established.[2,4,10] Furthermore, if a patient is heavily medicated with these drugs, the warning signs and symptoms that convulsions are eminent will usually be masked.

■Preparations and Precautions Prior to Regional Block: Although regional anesthesia is less likely to result in a catastrophe than general anesthesia, its conduct, particularly for a major regional block procedure (epidural, spinal, and peripheral nerve block), should be the same as for general anesthesia.

☐Start intravenous fluids. Simply placing a plastic catheter needle ("heparin lock") in a vein is not enough, for it may become obstructed; and even if it is patent when a systemic toxic reaction occurs, precious seconds or minutes can be lost in attaching fluids to it.

☐Resuscitative equipment and drugs must be readied for use and injection within five to ten seconds of onset of a reaction.

☐Preoxygenate the patient. This may be debatable, but it does assure immediate availability of oxygen.

☐Attach a blood pressure cuff and electrocardioscope.

☐Have present one additional person who is capable of doing effective cardiopulmonary resuscitation.

☐Add epinephrine to the local anesthetic solution to lower plasma levels of the local anesthetic drug and counter the myocardial depression of local anesthetic drugs. A 1:200,000 epinephrine content (0.1 mg epinephrine per 20 ml of local anesthetic solution) is optimal, but 0.25 mg of epinephrine is not exceeded. Otherwise an epinephrine reaction may result.

☐Aspirate for blood or cerebrospinal fluid.

☐Administer a test dose. Many anesthesiologists do not inject a test dose of local anesthetic drugs, particularly when using a single-injection technique, for numerous rational reasons.[11-13] Others employ ineffective test doses.[14-17] An effective test dose should be given prior to epidural or caudal block, as well as peripheral nerve blocks of the head and neck.

Prior to interscalene brachial plexus block, stellate ganglion block, and other head and neck blocks, 1 to 2 ml (depending on the concentration) of plain solutions of local anesthetic drugs will immediately indicate an inadvertent intravascular or subarachnoid injection. Contrarily, to achieve this result for lumbar epidural or caudal block, the test dose must contain 0.015 mg of epinephrine (Adrenalin), that is, the amount contained in 3 ml of a 1:200,000 solution, and a milligram dose of the local anesthetic drugs which produces conclusive evidence of spinal anesthesia--for example, 45 to 50 mg of lidocaine (Xylocaine[*]) or mepivacaine (Carbocaine[*]), or 12 to 15 mg of bupivacaine.[18] A 3 ml test dose of a solution containing these ingredients will produce a recognizable epinephrine reaction within 45 seconds, indicating an intravascular injection, and spinal block within two minutes if injected subarachnoidally. Signs and symptoms of these in the unmedicated patient will speak for themselves. The moderately medicated patient, however, must be monitored with the electrocardioscope, preferably with a heart-rate indicator, for a sustained rise in heart rate within 45 seconds from the epinephrine. After two minutes have elapsed, the buttock(s) is pinched with an instrument (Allis forceps) to reveal presence or absence of sensation.[18]

While a test dose as detailed will indicate the possibility of a systemic toxic reaction from the therapeutic dose of a local anesthetic drug intravascularly, it is worthless in indicating the possibility of such a reaction from absorption. Also, beta adrenergic blockers such as propranolol (Inderal[*]) negate the increase in heart rate caused by epinephrine, and when the patient is taking these drugs, other signs and symptoms of an intravascular injection must be monitored, such as an increase in blood pressure.[18]

☐Meticulous monitoring of the cardiovascular and respiratory systems should be routine following injection of a local anesthetic drug, a narcotic, or a tranquilizer. The patient should be monitored at least every 15 to 30 seconds for the first five minutes, then at least at five-minute intervals.

☐Keep an accurate record of events.

■Treatment of Systemic Toxicity: This depends on the signs and symptoms, but within five to ten seconds of the onset, the patient must be ventilated with oxygen. When systemic toxicity from a local anesthetic drug occurs, our dictum is, "Reach for the mask, not the syringe or endotracheal tube."

☐Self-limiting convulsions: The treatment which we have used for 38 years to resolve more than 135 self-limiting convulsions and which has avoided in all those patients cardiac arrest, brain damage, and death is as follows, and is performed in sequence as numbered.

---

[*]Registered trademark.

1. Establish a patent airway. Suction vomitus and place an oral airway if necessary, but do not attempt to intubate. We have yet to intubate a patient with a self-limiting convulsion.
2. Ventilate with oxygen.
3. If necessary, administer a drug(s) to make ventilation easier (succinylcholine 50 to 60 mg, diazepam 5 to 10 mg, thiopental 75 to 100 mg). Give the drug intravenously as a bolus and expect apnea. No one should inject a local anesthetic drug unless he/she can direct and execute efficient cardiopulmonary resuscitation.

☐Cardiac arrest: In the 38 years that I have been doing regional block, no cardiac arrests have occurred during or after a systemic toxic reaction to a local anesthetic drug. Nonetheless, ventilation with oxygen, manual systole, drugs to treat arrest, and blood gas determinations to avoid overventilation is the treatment.[17]

☐Arrhythmias: Bradycardia is treated by ventilation with oxygen and by injecting 0.1 to 0.2 mg of epinephrine intravenously. Other arrhythmias (bigeminy, etc.) respond to ventilation with oxygen and sedation with diazepam 2.5 to 5 mg or thiopental 50 to 75 mg intravenously. Whether 50 mg of lidocaine should be used is open to question.

☐Immediate cardiopulmonary collapse ("anaphylactic shock") is treated by cardiopulmonary resuscitation.

☐Sustained convulsions lasting two and one-half to three and one-half hours (only two reported in the literature) have been effectively treated by ventilation, anesthetizing the patient until signs of convulsions disappear, intubating, and keeping the patient anesthetized until the convulsions terminate.[19-21]

■Information Required to Evaluate a Catastrophe from Systemic Toxicity: Prior to "labeling" bupivacaine, etidocaine, or any other drug as a cardiotoxic drug, as has previously been done, the following must be known: (1) the circumstances under which the block was performed; (2) the interval between the start of convulsions and the initiation of emergency therapy; (3) the therapeutic endeavors; and (4) the sequence of therapeutic endeavors.[1]

NEUROTOXICITY OF LOCAL ANESTHETIC DRUGS

Reported cases of neuropathy from solutions of chloroprocaine (Nesacaine-CE; CE indicates for caudal and epidural block), as well as theories as to why they have occurred, have resulted in many anesthesiologists, including us, discontinuing the use of chloroprocaine until the specific etiology is determined and eliminated.[22-29] Whether the neuropathy is a result of the milligram dose of chloroprocaine, the low pH (acidity) of its solutions, the 2 mg/ml of sodium bisulfite (antioxidizing agent), or a combination of these, remains unknown.

Pennwalt Laboratories, distributors of chloroprocaine, contends that it is no more neurotoxic than other local anesthetic drugs.[30,31] Pennwalt states: "Solutions of Nesacaine and Nesacaine-CE do not injure nervous tissue and are not irritating to other tissues in the concentrations recommended."[32] Nonetheless, until the cause of the neuropathy is discovered and eliminated, anyone using chloroprocaine and having a neuropathy result may run the risk of being accused of negligence. For example, in 1947 Dr. Graham had two cases of paraplegia resulting from the use of ampules of drugs for spinal anesthesia that had been soaked in "carbolic disinfectant." The following quotation is from the British Medical Journal report of the 1954 review decision of Lord Justice Denning in the case against Dr. Graham.[33]

"We must not look at this 1947 accident with 1954 spectacles," said his lordship. "The judge acquitted Dr. Graham of negligence, and we should uphold his decision. Never again, it was to be hoped, would such a thing happen. It was the extraordinary accident of these two men which first disclosed the danger. Nowadays, it would be negligence not to realize the danger, but it was not then."

Should the acidity of the chloroprocaine solution prove to be the etiology of the neuropathies, injecting a solution with a low pH can be avoided with other local anesthetic drugs. We use only plain solutions of local anesthetic drugs from single-dose ampules and vials. The pHs of these solutions are 4.5 or above (Table 2). If epinephrine is desirable in the solution, we add it immediately before injection. Doing so does not alter the pH of the local anesthetic solution (Table 2).[34] We do not inject commercially prepared solutions with epinephrine.

Table 2

LOCAL ANESTHETIC SOLUTIONS: pH

	pH*		
Drug	Plain	Epinephrine Added by DCM▲	Commercially Prepared Solutions with Epinephrine
■ bupivacaine (Marcaine®)	5.7	5.7	3.8
■ chloroprocaine (Nesacaine®)	2.9	2.9	
■ etidocaine (Duranest®)	4.5	4.5	3.8
■ lidocaine (Xylocaine®)	6.3	6.3	3.8
■ mepivacaine (Carbocaine®)	5.5	5.5	
■ prilocaine (Citanest®)	6.5	6.5	

*Determined by Beckman model 3560 digital pH meter.
▲Daniel C. Moore.

COMPUTED TOMOGRAPHY

CT (computed tomography) has been proven to be the most accurate method of insuring correct needle placement when performing therapeutic blocks, particularly alcohol celiac plexus block (Figure 1).

With CT the precise position of the points of the needles can be determined in relationship to the following anatomical structures, which it visualizes: (1) the aorta and vena cava; (2) the subarachnoid or epidural space; (3) the kidney; (4) the renal pelvis; (5) the crura of the diaphragm; (6) the pleura and lung; and (7) other vital structures. Furthermore, the spread of the 50 ml of 50 percent alcohol can be documented, if the solution contains the following: (1) 25 ml of absolute alcohol; (2) 18 ml of 0.75 percent bupivacaine; and (3) 7 ml of iothalamate meglumine (Conray).[35]

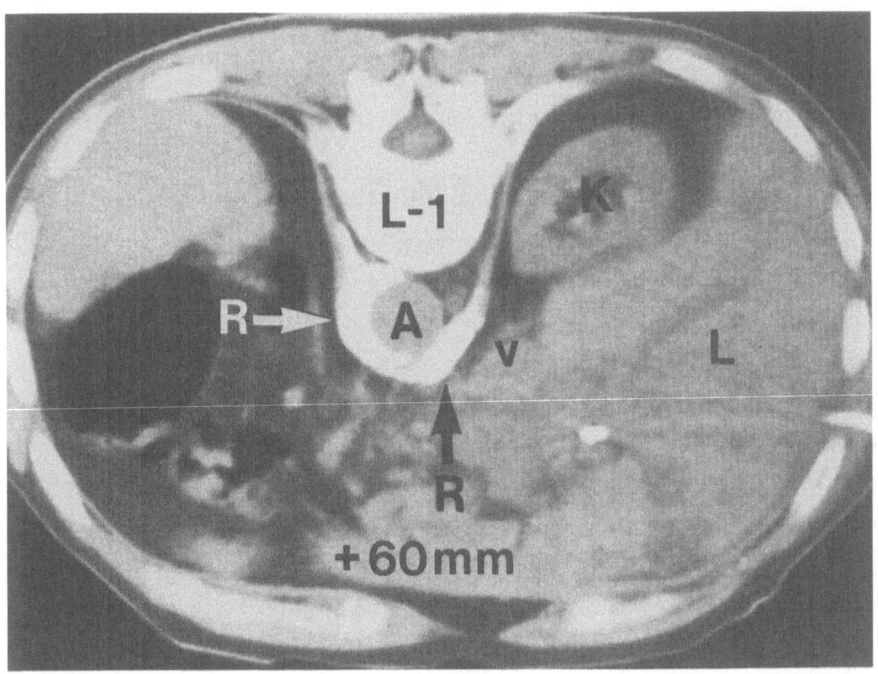

FIGURE 1. L-1, first lumbar vertebra; K, kidney; A, aorta; v, vena cava; R, radiopaque alcohol solution; + 60 mm, scan taken 60 millimeters above hubs of needles.

INTERCOSTAL NERVE BLOCK

Block of the intercostal nerve(s) results in the highest blood levels of the local anesthetic drug which occur more rapidly than when a comparable dose is injected for epidural block (lumbar or caudal), brachial plexus block, or sciatic, femoral, lateral femoral cutaneous, and/or obturator nerve blocks.[36,37] This has been shown to occur as a result of the extensive spread of the drug in the costal groove of the rib and in the internal intercostal muscles.[38] Also, this and another study have confirmed that the optimal site for injecting the intercostal nerves is at the angle of the rib.[38,39] These two articles disagree about the number of nerves blocked by each injection. Further studies in corpses (cadavers) confirmed that only the intercostal nerve of the groove injected is bathed by the local anesthetic solution.[40]

WHAT'S NEW WITH SUBARACHNOID (SPINAL) BLOCK?

A study of 435 patients compared the anesthetic properties (onset, duration, quality of analgesia, etc.) of bupivacaine and tetracaine, using 7.5 and 12 mg of each.[41] In those investigations other variables were studied, which showed the following.

■Cephalalgia: In 218 of these patients in whom a Greene point needle was used, no cephalalgia from the dura tap resulted. Sixty-two of these patients were males and 156 were females. Their ages ranged from 15 to over 60, with 168 being under the age of 50. The Greene point needle differs from other needles in that its bevel has no cutting edges. Therefore, as with the pencil-point needle, it spreads rather than cuts the longitudinal fibers of the dura.

■Hypotension: The larger the dose of a local anesthetic drug, the greater the incidence of hypotension.

■Height, Weight, and Dosage in Relationship to Dermatome Level: Using the same dosage and the stepwise regression test of significance, and weight divided by height squared, the results showed that the heavier the patient of comparable height, the higher the dermatome level of analgesia ($p < 0.005$).

■Epinephrine Added to the Local Anesthetic Solution: Solutions with epinephrine resulted in dermatome levels four dermatomes higher than those without epinephrine ($p < 0.025$).

■Accuracy of Needle Placement: A line drawn between the iliac crests crosses either the spinous process of the fourth lumbar vertebra or the interspace between the spinous processes of the fourth and fifth lumbar vertebrae. This was used as a guide for placing the spinal needle in the second lumbar interspace in 100 consecutive patients. Roentgenograms of needle placement were taken, and in 81, 14, and five patients the needle was in the second, first, and third lumbar interspace, respectively.

Misplacement of the needle occurred in the short and/or obese patient. In these patients, what we determined to be the second lumbar interspace was in most instances the first lumbar interspace.

REFERENCES

1. Albright GA: Cardiac arrest following regional anesthesia with etidocaine or bupivacaine. Anesthesiology 51:285-286, 1979.
2. Moore DC: Administer oxygen first in the treatment of local anesthetic-induced convulsions (Correspondence). Anesthesiology 53:346-347, 1980.
3. Orringer CE, Eustace JC, Wunch CD, Gardner LB: Natural history of lactic acidosis after grand-mal seizures. N Engl J Med 15:796-799, 1977.
4. Moore DC, Crawford RD, Scurlock JE: Severe hypoxia and acidosis following local anesthetic-induced convulsions. Anesthesiology 53:259-260, 1980.
5. Tatum AL, Atkinson AJ, Collins KH: Acute cocaine poisoning, its prophylaxis and treatment in laboratory animals. J Pharmacol Exp Ther 26:325-335, 1925.
6. Tatum AL, Collins KH: Acute cocaine poisoning and its treatment in monkeys (Macacus Rhesus). Arch Intern Med 38:405-409, 1926.
7. deJong RH, Heavner JE: Diazepam prevents and aborts lidocaine convulsions in monkeys. Anesthesiology 41:226-230, 1974.
8. Moore DC, Bridenbaugh LD: Oxygen: The antidote for systemic toxic reactions from local anesthetic drugs. JAMA 174:842-847, 1960.
9. Moore DC, deJong RH: Toxic effects of local anesthetics (Letters). JAMA 240:434, 1978.
10. Moore DC, Balfour RI, Fitzgibbons D: Convulsive arterial plasma levels of bupivacaine and the response to diazepam therapy. Anesthesiology 50:454-456, 1979.
11. Bromage PR: Epidural Anesthesia. Philadelphia: WB Saunders Company, 1978, pp 201-202.
12. Edde RR, Deutsch S: Cardiac arrest after interscalene brachial plexus block. Anesth Analg 55:446-447, 1977.
13. Hodgkinson R, Husain FJ: Epidural test dose in obstetrics (Letter). Anesth Analg 59:811, 1980.
14. Datta S, Corke BC, Alper MH, Brown WU, Ostheimer GW, Weiss JB: Epidural anesthesia for cesarean section: A comparison of bupivacaine, chloroprocaine and etidocaine. Anesthesiology 52:48-51, 1980.
15. Fargas-Babjak F, McChesney J, Morison DH: The efficacy of bupivacaine 0.75 per cent as an epidural test dose. Can Anaesth Soc J 27:500-501, 1980.
16. Schweitzer SA: Avoiding intravascular injections during epidural anesthesia. Anesthesiology 53:81, 1980.
17. Prentiss JE: Cardiac arrest following caudal anesthesia. Anesthesiology 50:51-53, 1979.
18. Moore DC: The necessary ingredients of a test dose prior to epidural or caudal block. Anesthesiology 53:S214, 1980.
19. Van Dongen LGR, Glientenberg H: A case of toxicity to excessive "Carbocaine" with probable reactivity of rheumatic disease. S. Afr Med J 35:73-76, 1961.
20. Moore DC: Regional Block, 4th ed. Springfield IL: Charles C Thomas, 1965, pp 23-24.
21. Moore, DC: Complications of regional anesthesia, in Bonica JJ (ed): Regional Anesthesia: Recent Advances and Current Status. Philadelphia: FA Davis Company, 1969, p 226.
22. Covino BG, Marx GF, Finster M, Zsigmond EK: Prolonged sensory/motor deficits following inadvertent spinal anesthesia. Anesth Analg 59:399-400, 1980.

23. Ravindran RS, Bond VK, Tasch MD, Gupta CD, Leurssen TG: Prolonged neural blockade following regional analgesia with 2-chloroprocaine. Anesth Analg 59:446-451, 1980.

24. Reisner LS, Hochman BN, Plumer MH: Persistent neurologic deficit and adhesive arachnoiditis following intrathecal 2-chloroprocaine injection. Anesth Analg 59:452-454, 1980.

25. Friedman G, DeFazio C: Prolonged neural blockade following regional anesthesia with 2-chloroprocaine. Anesth Analg 59:810, 1980.

26. Barsa JE, Batra M, Fink BR: Prolonged neural blockade following regional anesthesia with 2-chloroprocaine. Anesth Analg 59:810-811, 1980.

27. McLeskey CH: pH of local anesthetic solutions. Anesth Analg 59:892-893, 1980.

28. Gibbs CP, Munson ES: Local anesthetic toxicity (Letter). Anesth Analg 59:955, 1980.

29. Reisner LS: Nesacaine is out. Newletter Society for Obstetrics and Perinatology 12:6, 1981.

30. Kane RE: Neurologic deficits following epidural and spinal anesthesia. Anesth Analg 60:150-161, 1981.

31. Govier WM: Cytoxicity of local anesthetics (Letter). Anesth Analg 60:168-169, 1981.

32. Physician Desk Reference. Oradell, NJ: Medical Economics Company, 1981, p 1397.

33. Medicine and law: Spinal anaesthesia. Lancet 2:1089-1090, 1953.

34. Moore DC: The chloroprocaine (Nesacaine) story: 1952-1980 (to be published).

35. Moore DC, Bush WH, Burnett LL: Celiac plexus block: A roentgenographic anatomic study of technique and spread of solution in humans and corpses. Anesth and Analg 1981 (June issue).

36. Moore DC, Mather LE, Bridenbaugh PO, Bridenbaugh LD, Balfour RI, Lysons DF, Horton WG: Arterial and venous plasma levels of bupivacaine following epidural and intercostal nerve blocks. Anesthesiology 45:39-45, 1976.

37. Moore DC, Mather LE, Bridenbaugh PO, Bridenbaugh LD, Balfour RI, Lysons DF, Horton WG: Arterial and venous plasma levels of bupivacaine following peripheral nerve block. Anesth Analg 55:763-768, 1976.

38. Moore DC, Bush W, Scurlock JE: Intercostal nerve block: A roentgenographic anatomic study of technique and absorption of solution in humans. Anesth Analg 59:815-825, 1980.

39. Nunn JF, Slavin G: Posterior intercostal nerve block for pain relief after cholecystectomy. Br J Anaesth 52:253-260, 1980.

40. Moore DC: Intercostal nerve block: Spread of India ink injected into the rib's costal groove. Br J Anaesth 1981 (April issue).

41. Moore DC: Spinal anesthesia: Bupivacaine compared with tetracaine. Anesth Analg 59:743-750, 1980.

INDEX

BOERHAAVE SERIES
FOR POSTGRADUATE
MEDICAL EDUCATION

1. Hemker HC, Loeliger EA, Veltkamp JJ, eds: Human blood coagulation. Biochemistry, clinical investigation, therapy. 1969. ISBN 90-6021-008-5
2. Goslings WRO, ed: Diseases of the gastro-intestinal tract. Some diagnostic, therapeutic and fundamental aspects. 1970. ISBN 90-6021-011-5
3. Haas JH de, Hemker HC, Snellen HA, eds: Ischaemic heart disease. 1970. ISBN 90-6021-012-3
4. Gevers RH, Ruys JH, eds: Physiology and pathology in the perinatal period. 1971. ISBN 90-6021-100-6
5. Elkerbout F, Thomas P, Zwaveling A, eds: Cancer chemotherapy. *Out of print*
6. Stoelinga GBA, Van der Werff ten Bosch JJ, eds: Normal and abnormal development of brain and behaviour. 1971. ISBN 90-6021-099-9
7. Spierdijk J, Feldman SA, eds: Anaesthesia and pharmaceutics. 1972. ISBN 90-6021-125-1
8. Snellen HA, Hemker HC, Hugenholtz PG, van Bemmel JH, eds: Quantitation in cardiology. 1972. ISBN 90-6021-139-1
9. Feldman SA, Leigh JM, Spierdijk J, eds: Measurement in anaesthesia. 1974. ISBN 90-6021-203-7
10. Hemker HC, Veltkamp JJ, eds: Prothrombin and related coagulation factors. 1975. ISBN 90-6021-236-3
11. Went LN, Vermeij-Keers C, van der Linden AGJM, eds: Early diagnosis and prevention of genetic diseases. 1975. ISBN 90-6021-237-1
12. Spierdijk J, Feldman SA, Mattie H, eds: Anaesthesia and pharmacology. With a special section on professional hazards. 1976. ISBN 90-6021-294-0
13. van Mierop LHS, Oppenheimer-Dekker A, Bruins CLDC, eds. Embryology and teratology of the heart and the great arteries. Conducting system; transposition of the great arteries; ductus arteriosus. 1978. ISBN 90-6021-424-2
14. de Wolff FA, Mattie H, Breimer DD, eds: Therapeutic relevance of drug assays. 1979. ISBN 90-6021-443-9
15. Keirse MJNC, Anderson ABM, Bennebroek Gravenhorst J, eds: Human parturition. 1979. ISBN 90-6021-445-5
16. van Oosterom AT, Muggia FM, Cleton FJ, eds: Therapeutic progress in ovarian cancer, testicular cancer and the sarcomas. 1980. ISBN 90-6021-452-8
17. van den Tweel JG, Taylor CR, Bosman FT, eds: Malignant lymphoproliferative diseases. 1980. ISBN 90-6021-451-X
18. Welvaart K, Blumgart LH, Kreuning J, eds: Colorectal Cancer. 1980. ISBN 90-6021-465-X
19. Daems WT, Burger EH, Afzelius BA, eds: Cell biological aspects of disease. The plasma membrane and lysosomes. 1981. ISBN 90-6021-466-8
20. Pauwels EK, Schütte HE, Taconis WK, Ell PJ, eds: Bone scintigraphy. 1981. ISBN 90-6021-476-5
21. Wenink ACG, Oppenheimer-Dekker A, Moulaert A, eds: Ventricular septum of the heart. 1981. ISBN 90-247-486-2
22. Keirse MJNC, Bennebroek Gravenhorst JJ, van Lith DAF, Embrey MP, eds: Second trimester pregnancy termination. 1982. ISBN 90-247-490-0
23. Spierdijk J, Feldman SA, Mattie H, Stanley TH, eds: Developments in drugs used in anaesthesia. 1981. ISBN 90-247-492-7